POWER COUPLING

POWER coupling

Coming Together When Life is Falling Apart

KATHERINE MCCLELLAND

NEW YORK

LONDON • NASHVILLE • MELBOURNE • VANCOUVER

Power Coupling
Coming Together When Life is Falling Apart

Published in New York, New York, by Morgan James Publishing in partnership with Difference Press. Morgan James is a trademark of Morgan James, LLC. www.MorganJamesPublishing.com

ISBN 9781642794854 paperback
ISBN 9781642794861 eBook
ISBN 9781642795882 audiobook
Library of Congress Control Number: 2019901526

Cover Design by:
Rachel Lopez
www.r2cdesign.com

Interior Design by:
Christopher Kirk
www.GFSstudio.com

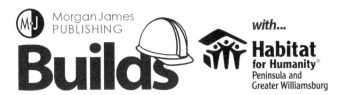

Morgan James is a proud partner of Habitat for Humanity Peninsula and Greater Williamsburg. Partners in building since 2006.

Get involved today! Visit
MorganJamesPublishing.com/giving-back

Coming Home to You

At the

    Edge of the Dream,

        throw yourself

all the way

          In.

CEO. Mother. Lover. Wife.

      Happy Mama. Happy Life.

Dedication

This book is dedicated to the work of Spirit in the world to unite us as One and draw us nearer each other in our hearts each day.

To my mother who gave the world everything she had to give, living every day fully with a heart of a true adventurer, she lived her life in service and love. She was an inspiration to many as she forged her own way. She has given me strength.

To the powerful women who have given myself and many others the tools with which to heal and empower themselves, whom I myself have come to know and love; and who have all contributed to this book through my adaptations of their teachings – all have conspired to teach me and guide me so that I now have access to creativity and power within to share with you – in deepest gratitude and with special kudos for healing and tools of growth to Mary Hulnick, Kathlyn Hendricks, Byron Katie, and to the men who have stood with them in partnership, Ron Hulnick, Gay Hendricks, and Stephen Mitchell (all accomplished men in their own right) – and specifically for this book, special recognition to Alison Armstrong for supplying me with a new set of tools for partnership, many of which are adapted and shared in my own way with her permission here, and to her husband, co-conspirator, and partner Greg and their fishbowl partnership learning laboratory that I and many others have learned so much from – and to all women everywhere in their devotion to their wholeness are healing themselves and this planet through their dedication to their full expression of themselves as the power of love – and to the men who love and support them too.

To Jack Ma and the inspiration of LQ.

And to Daron, Tucker, and Brooks for being an invitation and inspiration to be the best human being I can be each day since I have had them in my life, and for the love and forgiveness in them that has made it all worthwhile.

Table of Contents

LQ: Love Intelligence: Part 3 –
         How to Get What You Need from Everyone. . 107

Author's Note

The process of writing this book has been magical and mysterious. I set out to write a book that was based in my past experience and share with you how my life journey became easier and joyful for me when I grounded myself in my life from a different source, and found my way home.

The Universe had different plans. The entire time I have been writing this book I have had to prove myself as committed to these principles or I would never have gotten this book done. This book reflects my authentic journey. I have walked this book in my life each day as I have written this book with you in my heart knowing if I could handle what I was up to, I could trust that you could too.

The entire time I have been writing this book I have been also holding space for and assisting with my 95-year-old mother's declining health. It has been a full-on challenge to hold both and the rest of life as well – this experience has guided my writing. This is the culmination of the meta point of the book – having a full life invites us to make a choice to either be to be hyper vigilant, tense and irritable, attempting to control everything, or to be calm and aware and choosing our attention moment to moment. If we choose the latter we can attend to our full lives with an easeful grace and without missing what is most important to us in each moment of each day.

I am starting with gratitude to all those who supported me in allowing and trusting right along with me, ensuring that I know them as my sacred circle, and the Universe for all the grace you have granted me in this process. And to my mother, Frances McClelland, for this final lesson of love.

Just as the final edit of this book was due, my mother died. I was there. Despite my book deadlines, I was there.

And now I realize why I needed to write this book – in the past, in my overwhelm, I very likely would have missed these last moments with my mother. But because as I wrote this book I had to impeccably live into what I was teaching, I was given a miracle. I want this same miraculous life available to you. If you have the time or inclination, I offer my newest experience of grace below.

The night before my mother died, I was sitting at home facing a very big book deadline for 6 o'clock the next morning and I had a long way to go. I had a sudden nudge to call my mother. As I did so, I was hoping that maybe I would get away with a ten-minute phone call, just see how she was and to reassure myself that the caregiver was tending to her needs, and then get back to work. When I asked my mother how her day was, instead of her standard recent response, "I just keep on keeping on, did some crosswords, ate some lunch," she said, "I don't know, today was different. I sat in my chair and thought about my life a lot." Something, maybe the tone of her voice and her choice to spend the day sitting in quiet rumination, maybe something deeper, spurred me out of my chair to her door. Within two minutes of my arrival we were immersed in a full-on crisis as my mother had some sort of heart or mind event that began the end of her life. I was there to breathe with her, to hold her in her fear, to reassure her, to give her the morphine that would bring her relief. I was there. And I was there until she died. Long after 6 a.m. No final draft turned in. I just trusted that it was going to be okay. I made my choice. I was committed to being there for my mother. Period.

Except of course, I needed to take care of me too.

In the later morning, having not slept much and needing some care myself, I went home and slept for a couple of hours, showered, and came back. She was stable through the night and into the early morning. Once I was back, I got in bed and talked to her, sang her a few lullabies, and snuggled up. She was no longer conscious and I had no idea what to expect. And then in the middle of the day, in a very unassuming way, she sweetly and elegantly took a gentle last breath and was gone.

I am so grateful for the way I live my life that I now know how to stay present and that I have learned to listen. The intuition that guided me to pick up the phone to call in that moment was not strong but it was there, and I followed it. Then again to pause in the space of my deadline, to really hear the significance of her words amidst it, to experience my intuition again, heed its call, propelling me into action to her side, this will make all the difference in my own life. My grief will be mine and unique, but it will not carry the sadness of having missed that moment of her fear and pain. I was there. And now, I am again committed even more to living my life in tune with mySelf in such a way as to even in my full life, to be able to hear when I am being called to give comfort, kindness or for direction for my day. I want that for you too. I am in awe of the knowing beyond knowing and I celebrate my ability to be connected, present, and available to that moment, to that divine direction. I know that what comes first in my life is always in flux and to know that in my listening I will find my way, amidst what could be chaos, to the highest calling of love, that is my great joy.

This is the gift I am attempting to give each of you. I hope you will accept it. It isn't easy, but what is? I am so grateful for you here investing in yourself. You are beautiful blessings in my life, already.

Be well, fly free, and come home to you.

CHAPTER 1

Signing up for the Dream

When you signed up for a perfect life, could you ever imagine that this was what it was going to look like?

Life was just going to be idyllic and beautiful and when the hard things did come up, well, you would meet them together, talking and agreeing on a plan and then jumping in to resolve the challenges and immediately feeling happy to jump back into your regular daily wonderful life. You could handle anything with grace and love and a lot of delicious sex.

And it went okay for the first couple of years – the first baby, the first forays into work and life. Your jobs were interesting and demanding and manageable, you worked out, went to dinner, had vacations, relied on your reliable help, were connected, and your romantic life was sexy and fun. You had lots of great friends, bought the house that you loved. Things were rolling. You were happy.

And now, you realize, it has crept up on you.

You are not happy anymore. Everything that was supposed to fall into place is starting to feel like it is falling apart instead.

Work was supposed to be a great job where you were fully expressed, honored, and respected, treated like the queen that you are, contributing fully from your special genius and acknowledged and appreciated for it.

As work became more intense, as you got more successful, there are now meetings all the time, crises and client needs that have to be handled on weekends and evenings. In many ways, work has taken over. You love your work but have lost some perspective or something. You don't know what is motivating you, but sometimes it feels like work is becoming more important to you than your family or your husband.

You really don't want to have this out of balance. It is costing you your home life and being there with your husband and kids. But, you do want this career. You want to be successful. And you want it to fit into your whole beautiful life. You need more hours in a day!

At home, it was to be all domestic bliss, beautiful well-behaved kids who were ready and glad to see you when you got home, and delightedly scampered off to play alone or peacefully with each other when you needed to kick your shoes off and have a martini with your husband. Their future was bright. Perfect schools for your kids, your property values would just increase, and your kids would be happy and choose lives where they would make you so proud – engineer, doctor, well, even artists or actors as long as they were successful and happy.

You added another child and as they grow up their needs are getting bigger and less easily solved (and then there is the sibling thing …). And your kids, they seem to be in a constant state of neediness, and they are showing signs of having issues that are bigger than you can handle at school. You are providing everything for them but nothing you do for them seems to be making a difference.

Ideally in your perfect picture, there would be one helper who would be able to handle all the needs of the family, of the children, shopping, meals and well, all the things Suzy's mother did (but your mother definitely didn't) keeping the house running calmly and organized to your specifications. She would know just how to raise the kids and perfectly manage a household. She would have perfect manners, never be out of sorts, and be helpful and ready to change direction whenever you needed her to. She would start with you and stay with you all the way until your kids went off to college and, she would have holidays with you and share in your family gatherings for the rest of your children's lives.

That is not the reality. Even when it was good and somewhat manageable, it was always a struggle to manage your helper while she managed your lives. And now she doesn't seem to be carrying her weight the way she was before. She is overwhelmed and making things harder on you. She doesn't seem to do things with the same grace as she used to and she seems unhappy and disgruntled a lot. She seems skittish and unsure of herself and a bit too easily cajoled by the kids. And you can't afford to let her go, so you are stuck with each other. You are both suffering from that.

And your marriage, your beautiful, blissful marriage. He was the guy. He was going to make it happen. And you were going to fall deeper and deeper in love every day. You were going to be the woman of his dreams and he would have no eyes for other women. You would share your beautiful family, enjoy each other fully, share in each other's successes, champion each other when things were tough, and sit back and enjoy your children growing up around you. You would have beautiful family vacations where everyone was happy and contented to love the moments and come back cheerful and refreshed from whatever adventures you chose that day.

You and your husband would have plenty of time to connect and stay sexually deeply connected, enjoy each other's bodies as both of you took the time and focus to stay in great shape and as beautiful as you were that perfect day of your wedding.

Your husband is less attentive; you aren't taking as good care of yourselves anymore. You are exhausted after vacations and your bodies are paying the price of your lives. You are losing interest in your sex life, and there is just never any time for anything you want anymore.

You could not be less interested in sex if your life depended on it. You are not as healthy. Even though you look okay in clothes, you hate to show your body. You have had a couple of kids and you know things are just not the same. You are not looking the way you want to be admired and desired. You definitely think your husband could lose a bit of "baby weight," too. You are starting to notice other men, to be honest, and you see him looking around, too. There are plenty of women who would be happy to sleep with him, you are sure. You just can't anymore. You don't know what is wrong with you. You are exhausted and running around, just barely keeping your head above water – you are supposed to be sexy and inviting, too? How can he expect that? He says he doesn't care if you are perfect or in shape, he just wants to have sex, but you just can't. You don't want to. You only see yourself as undesirable. You never realized what this life would do to your body and your self.

Your health is slipping. You are finding yourself reaching for coffee, sugar, and anything that will prop you up. You haven't worked out in months and can't even make yourself go when you have the time. It isn't really that bad yet, but you feel too embarrassed to go back and start again. You feel uncomfortable, but you guess it is better than feeling like you are going to freak out from the pressure. You want to be healthy, you want to feel good. You want to be flexible and strong as you age.

As your health changes, you see your face and hair, your beauty, changing too. You see lines from stress and worry, and see bags under and rings around your eyes. You are not sleeping well, so you look pasty and unrested. You don't want to lose your sense of youth and beauty, too. You've been buying all sorts of cosmetics and are thinking a lot about Botox and facelifts as you look at in the mirror in the morning. You want to feel beautiful as you step toward your forties. You want to see your beauty blossoming again. Nothing that you have tried, bought, or done is really helping yet.

And then there's wine. So, you have to have a drink or two at the end of the day… and maybe you have started having wine earlier, before the kids get home, to cope a little better, or if they are home, you'll sneak off to the bathroom and drink a quick glass to get a head start. You just can't take the constant pressure, you need some relief. It's better than you yelling at everyone at the end of the day.

You have not felt yourself for so long you don't even know if you are here anymore. You just go from one meeting to the next, one responsibility to the next, one nanny to the next … one school, one meal, one desperate breath. Sometimes you get into the car and burst into tears.

And now life is becoming a firestorm of irritability and frustration. No one is getting their needs met and everyone is suffering.

This out-of-control life is starting to take everything from you.

You were so sure you could do this. And you knew that no matter what anyone said, it was possible. Sure there would maybe be some leaner years in the beginning, but you would build your life and it would go smoothly in the direction of more resources to spend and care for yourselves with. You had all this to look forward to on your wedding day.

So how did you get so far from that wedding day, or even those first few years? How did you lose your way? You've seen it. You've seen where this can go – job lost, kids flailing, husband out and away a lot. Or even divorce. It happens a lot.

"I feel everything slipping away. Everything. I am terrified I am going to lose it all. I can't do that. I have planned this all so carefully. It is my dream. Now all I see is the nightmare."

This is the "losing-it-all" nightmare you worry about now, every day.

You may not be here yet, but you see yourself on the slide. Your system is stressed and you perceive that this nightmare is actually in your foreseeable future.

But let's step back and inventory: what is really happening?

You have no time for *you*. You aren't even sure that this is such a big deal in your life, but the yoga by yourself and the books for inspiration that you would read in the past would really keep you balanced and focused on getting your thoughts and yourself in the right place to support the life you want. You just don't have the inclination to find time for you anymore. There is just too much else to do. And really, this life is the life you chose, it is all for you. It is what you want, after all.

You used to love to plan your future in your mind and sometimes make collages or write poetry and feel into what you wanted your life to feel like, happy and pleasant and fun. You don't do these things anymore. You don't have the desire to go there for some reason.

Maybe you are just too burned out. You don't really see the point. You have no plans for your future, you are just trying to get through today. Your creativity feels like it has dried up and what you used to do doesn't give you the same pleasure anymore. You are focusing so much that you feel like your head is going to explode sometimes.

You feel like you need to figure this out. You need to do something to get all this chaos under control and reclaim your life.

You can see that this is not sustainable. If you don't pull it together you feel that there is a good chance that you are going to live your worst nightmare – you are going to lose your work and your husband, your kids are going to fall apart, and everything you have ever built is going to fall away.

And, you don't want to read about yourself or your kids or your husband on Facebook or hear the gossip at the club or see the averted eyes. You have lived through this with your friends.

You have a seminal moment and finally you get your own attention. And as you find yourself you think to yourself:

"This. Is. Not. Going. To. Happen. To. Me. It *stops* now."

That's why you are here.

That is why we are going to go on this journey together. I assure you, it does not have to slide into chaos, or be ignored until it all falls apart. Or blamed on someone else. Or given away to another woman. Or destroyed. Your life is yours. Seize the day.

And, you are right; it needs your attention, now.

I guarantee that if you take this on, deeply, fully, and with commitment, you will change what is not working, and you will give yourself the life of your dreams.

And, if you don't, if you keep looking away, coping, or entertaining yourself through what doesn't feel good, you will be giving it away. Think very hard before you do that.

Give your life the chance to prove to you that it is worthy of you, and yourself the chance to prove that you are worthy of your life. You are creating what you want, and that while you may have to tweak it, it is your life, and you can make it happen.

In this book, you will get the chance to sort out what you want, and how to get it. You will be invited to strengthen your values, your voice, your resolve, and your spirit, into having the space and the unlimited possibility to create from your joy and live, love, and have fun and power with your job, with your kids, and your husband every day. And you will have to do something different from what you are doing now to get there.

Chapter 2

Burnout on the Way

I left my first career in my late twenties. I literally walked out of my successful career on to the streets of NYC, jobless, a little nervous and exquisitely happy, thinking I would never look back and was leaving it all behind. And three years later, I went even further and left my whole life behind. My dog, my car, and whatever fit into it, I drove away and into the very different future I had now planned for myself.

I moved to a new life, new city, in many ways a new world. I worked hard, went back to school, lived through some challenging personal crises, and, was eventually ready for marriage, family, and the work of my dreams! In my mid-thirties, as I settled into my new career as a minister at a nonreligious Spiritual Center, I knew it! This was it.

It was everything I ever wanted. Part of my work was to be out in the community spreading goodwill and being involved in bringing heart to different community efforts. I served on boards of everything from green coalitions to nursery schools, co-founding an Interfaith Alliance to call the different religions together to talk about peace and conflict resolution and to create community-wide events that promoted healing and forgiveness and love. I was doing my part! The world was going to be a better place with me in it!

I had three kids at home many days. We were a blended family and I had two beautiful stepchildren (ages eleven and fourteen) and one little one (four) from my marriage. I loved all of them very much and was so happy to have them all around, and their friends!

My church was thriving, lots of friendly faces and people who came out to participate and be a part of our message of love, joy, peace, and personal responsibility.

Everything from Chapter 1 in this book was true for me. I married the man of my dreams with an idyllic image of what life was going to be like. We moved from the big city to the town everyone wants to live in, were settled in my dream home, my dream job. The kids were doing well, we had plenty of financial security. Everything was perfect, we could handle whatever came up - or so we thought.

And then the cracks started to show …

The first crack showed up in that my husband worked out of town, an hour and a half drive from our home (when there was no traffic). What had seemed so doable in our fantasy life, wasn't. He spent many long hours on freeways in Southern CA, leaving at 4:30 a.m. and arriving home after 7:30 many nights. This left him exhausted at the end of the day of working and driving, and left me to gather kids, take them places and provide meals, help and assist and care for them, exhausted too. And I loved them all so much that I wanted to do it all.

And then I was fully into my next chapter, as the Lead Minister in a spiritual center. I was certainly not thinking of my church as a business, but I had a lot to learn. I was thinking this was a spiritual job part time, graceful in and out, but I was wrong. I was running it full time, with a board of directors and a full congregation of "customers" to support. Outreach (marketing) and stewardship (sales), bottom line responsibilities and employees, people we were responsible for paying each Sunday – we were running a business. Two years into it I realized, I was the CEO *and* at the top of everyone's list for the prayer they needed. Holding both of those roles, along with parent and wife, was undoing me. The pressure was on.

The church was thriving and abundant with people and Spirit, but we never had enough money. From my earlier career, I started to think I understood what was needed. I buckled down and began to get more pragmatic and less, well, spiritual about the whole thing. I asked my husband to join me in the decision to donate my salary back to the church so we could pay other people for their contributions. I was okay, after all; my husband was making plenty for us to live on. In support of me, he agreed.

And then he lost his job.

As this was unfolding, my health started to fail. I had broken my arm and had a very challenging healing process. After a year with two surgeons whom one could easily argue made matters worse, I chose to take my healing seriously and went to a specialty clinic out of state to begin the healing over again. It was to take four more years and six more surgeries to complete, involving re-breaking both of my arm bones and replacing the tendons of my wrist/hand and getting fascia out of my thigh. And during that time, my general health was flagging, along with weight gain, no exercise, and little sex drive.

And then there was the exhaustion, and the fighting, and the blaming and the no sex and then the inevitable infidelity issues.

For Goodness sake, I was the Minister of Love and I could not love myself out of a paper bag no matter how hard I tried! All my relationships were in a shambles.

Oh No! How did we get here?

Now you know. I get it.

The hardest part for me about all of this was that I had few good skills that could really help with daily life at that time. We felt like we had our hands tied behind our backs. I was full of love and good intentions, but I was lost in the day-to-day reality of my life. We were trying to be loving but we just couldn't do anything like getting this right. We could not figure out what was wrong and any real way to fix it. We went to therapy for three years (didn't help), we prayed (didn't help), I went to spiritual retreats (didn't help), he went out with friends (didn't help), I went out with friends (didn't help). I had an emotional affair, he had the others. Not only was it too little, it was indeed too late.

Life was complete chaos. Complete chaos. Money collapsing, house milking us dry, surgeons/doctors and hospital bills reaching into high six figures. Work was pressing on me, our arguing was distressing the kids, the kids needed attention … we were all pressed to our limits and nothing was going well. We just finally gave up.

I don't want that for you.

Because my loss was so huge, the disaster so all-encompassing for me, I committed to find out how to never ever have myself or anyone else needlessly go down this kind of a road again. My work to get centered again was clear – to help myself first, and then help other people. Through my own experiences I began to see and map for others what needed to be in place in the beginning, to see the truth, not the fantasy, to support themselves in the truth, to be kind and fair and loving when things went wrong, to let go of the demands of perfection and to get back on track with more peace and joy in their lives. As we work through these things, things will change. Of course, they will – and that is precisely what you want. You want them to change, it's just that you want them to change in a good way. With what you can learn here, that is possible. And it will be up to you to do the work.

As I studied everything I could get my hands on for ten years, experimenting in my life and working with clients along the way, making integral changes in my own relationships, I have seen the power of the mindset and the skills I have learned. I have been helping clients change things in a good way since then. Every time a marriage is put on its right footing, every time someone is able to right their ship and get back the equilibrium that was lost, every time people find a way to get everything they want, I breathe a sigh of relief and let go a little more of whatever sadness has stayed with me from the experience as my whole life came crashing down. Each time I am of service to those who are struggling and help others find their way back, I breathe a little easier.

Now I do know what to do. Now, with all the study and experience I have had since then, I could tell you all of the places where this began in my marriage and my life, long before anything became obvious, anything already mentioned in this book. I can help. I can help you save your life, your career, your kids, and your marriage, in almost any stage.

As I was pulling together the strands of the work to share with my clients, I came across Jack Ma and his conversation about Love Quotient (LQ), also known as Love Intelligence. It occurred to me that his concepts of honor and respect as the basis for a love intelligence could serve as a framework in which to clarify my work.

I will digress a moment as I explain. I will introduce you to the concept of LQ as coined by Jack Ma (CEO/founder of Alibaba Group and self-made billionaire) and the ingredients of LQ as it pertains to partnerships. It is the final link to an absolute intelligence potential we all carry within us. In the US, we are all familiar with IQ. We are less familiar with EQ (Emotional Intelligence Quotient) but it is well accepted, and BQ (Body Intelligence Quotient) is breaking ground and is more and more accepted. To that we add LQ, which is generally not well defined or well accepted yet.

LQ is not a glorified EQ. It is not a different emotionally-based system or a spiritualized BQ, or a softer IQ. It has elements of all three, yet it provides its own addition to our understanding. It is your Love Intelligence. Love Intelligence is sourced in consciousness, and comes into our bodies and awareness through its intersection with these other intelligences. It provides a context of dignity of our humanity and, based in source, serves to bind all the other intelligence systems in our humanity, in our love. Inherent in it is that it is a part of everything, a component that has been missing from our understanding of how to relate to life, ourselves, and each other in life.

Your Love Intelligence is already in you, integrated in the deepest sense of who you are. It has its roots in honor and respect, two of the deepest capacities of Love. These two ingredients are absolutely necessary for thriving in human beings. We have needed a system that focuses us on the ways in which we carry our basic humanity within us and share that with each other. We will not become all that we can be, we will not reach our potential and solve the problems of our humanness without this. We must step beyond our intelligent but limited brains and into the larger system that supports our higher level of knowing. When we do, we will have access to extraordinary knowing, creativity, possibility, and compassion. In deference to Einstein, who has famously reminded us that we can't solve problems from within the level of consciousness where they were created, this LQ framework gives us access to the alternate level of consciousness where issues can be resolved.

I have created and will be sharing with you this journey to that higher mind. I will give you the tools to gain open access to the field that has within it the expanded consciousness far greater than our problem creating thinking mind. We will be traveling on what might be an unfamiliar road to you, to a higher mind based in a field of oneness, a wholistic system that connects everything to Itself. This field is where we experience our source as one with all in an expanded consciousness. This is where the roots of LQ are. This is how dramatically different this system is from the other intelligence quotients. This one begins in a universal intelligence and leads us directly to our deepest knowing, our most integrated intelligence, and the most powerful possibilities for solving our problems. In an effort to differentiate all of the different types of intelligence, LQ brings a context of the dignity of our humanity and, based in source, serves to ground all the other intelligence systems in our loving. It has as its roots an infinite intelligence. The BQ movement, which Kathlyn Hendricks co-founded, defined, and teaches with mastery is another powerful system of natural connection to ourselves. Her unique voice as a leader in that field is particularly important in increasing our awareness of our experience of reactivity and responsiveness and in accessing higher levels of knowing and consciousness through the body. Obviously we need IQ and our personal brain to participate, and EQ plays its part in the ease with which we facilitate our partnerships. The LQ system however is unique as it is universal and the basis of all of our humanity. It grounds in our truest selves and connects us with all other personal intelligences. It is the space that will give us back to our source, our humanity, and creates within us a world where peace, health, kindness, abundance, compassion, and wellbeing for ourselves, all beings, and this planet are available every day.

The one caveat is that from outside of this field, outside of the sense of wholeness and love in this field, we will not sense that it exists. We might rationally believe it, but to actually feel it, we must first choose to know that it is already there. You don't have to stake your life on it, but you will need to jump in and do the work before you have proof. This creates a dilemma; in order to be successful, you will need to choose to be curious and open as I am teaching you. In order to follow this path you will need to choose to trust that it is already there or at least be willing to play and trust me to guide you. Once you touch it you will know.

As we explore these concepts, I will be teaching you a system that I created with contribution from many sources. In this culture where all people thrive, we will be starting with you. You will learn the larger concepts and how to apply them in your life to make a difference for yourself, your loved ones, and in the world immediately. In each area, you will be given resources to make a difference in your partnerships and get the results you have wanted. Your overall experience of more giving and receiving, more love, more kindness, will result in a deeper sense of peace, compassion, joy, and partnerships that work. And while the specifics of what you want will look different in different areas of your life (business, home, husband, kids, friendships, and others), since they will all be based in your awareness of your Love Intelligence, they will bring you more wholeness, happiness, and peace everywhere.

If you really want results and not excuses, this book has a great plan for you. If you want the cutting edge newest framework (based in the oldest wisdom), and want to learn how to use the tools and get what you want with joy and without suffering, you are in the right place. I am not telling you the details of how we get there right now – that's for the next eight chapters – but the fact that we are going to be able to do this with no one sacrificing, no tears except for ones of healing and relief, and with everyone feeling good in the end?

That's priceless.

Would you like to be in love every day in your life? That is the result I play for every time. And I am happy to play for it with you.

LQ: Love Intelligence:
Part 1 –

WHAT IS THE SOURCE
OF YOUR LIFE?

CHAPTER 3

Our Adventure Begins with Source, Personal Culture, and Relational Partnerships

*I*n the case of David and Annie (names changed for sure), they had started where you and I started. We all had this idyllic fantasy that life was just always going to be beautiful for us, easy, and everything was going to work itself out without having to work on it or add more resources or look closely at ourselves.

The wedding was glorious, David and Annie glowing in their praise of each other, the bride in her beauty, the groom handsome, the shared children from their blended family in the wedding, happy and seemingly thriving with their new parent team.

She worked a lot. She had so much to do running the business that she had owned for twenty years. His job was important too, but he definitely had more flexibility to help with the kids. They had talked it out and tried to think of everything. They felt sure that it was going to be smooth sailing for them.

And, before they knew it, the kids were struggling and calling Annie at work. There were not enough hours in a day to get them all where they were supposed to be and cared for along the way. She felt like her work was suffering. Her employees didn't seem as happy, something she knew was very important to her, too.

There was a tension, the constant pressure on Annie to do more of the mom stuff, to show up to more of the kid stuff, but she had the main job. And, she even had the pressure from the inside more than the outside. She knew she was being judged by the other moms and by her circle for not showing up for her kids. And she now was a stepmom, too. It worried her a lot. She wanted to make sure that all the kids were covered. She would get tense and irritable about it.

And then her husband got laid off. It seemed perfectly simple, she thought. He would take care of the kids. Except that it did not work for him at all.

She tried to make David do things for the kids for her. He was a great dad, but he couldn't stand hanging out with a bunch of moms at functions or waiting for the kids to get out of a class. He said he would rather cut off a limb than stand there for five minutes… and he didn't think the kids needed so much coddling. His kids didn't need it so as far as he could see, it was her problem. This caused a lot of friction.

David and Annie came to see me, and so we began.

The first part of the process was to get very tactical. How do we best support this family in a way that works? We decided that they definitely needed more help, and that some of that help had to be of a professional caliber. A personal assistant/house manager was added so that the nanny could take care of the kids and not everything else.

We were able to work through a process of clarification for both David and Annie and they ended up with a very creative plan that they could both live with without sacrificing anything. In addition, while the nanny and house manager were good, both parents saw how important it was to the kids to actually have their parents there. They were able to make a plan and work together to make that happen as often as possible.

The process we engaged in was simple, but not easy. And it gave them a gift to pass on to the kids, too. It gave the kids a way to look at finding solutions that was respectful, and they even got the kids involved and made some deals about how everyone could assist in making these things happen more easily.

Before we were able to do this, we had to invite everyone into the idea that solving our problems by giving them to others without requesting support and getting an agreement is a recipe for disaster. Before I stepped in, David was starting to get depressed and was spending more and more time on the couch. That was also a point of tension. In Annie's mind, "What was he doing to help? He isn't even working."

As this process unfolds in uniquely respectful and honoring way for each individual, it leaves no room for forcing and/or manipulating others to bend to our will. That is a strategy that many people use unconsciously. It creates a lot of anger under the surface when we are trying to find ways to work together. We all manipulate each other differently; some of us use intimidation, some crying, some whining, some sex. When we really want our way, we will go to very great ends to get it. Think about this: when someone says no to you but you really want them to say yes, what do you do?

In another of our working sessions about each person's individual needs, the conversation inevitably touched on the topic of sex. The conversation started with Annie saying, "He wants sex all the time and I just don't get it." There was silence and tension as David breathed and processed his instruction to express himself fully, clearly, authentically, and vulnerably, to look deeply for what sex truly gave him. As David looked into Annie's eyes with his voice clearly shaking, he simply said to her, "Annie, when we make love you take me to God."

The room shivered. It was powerful truthful and deep expression of him. In that moment, with that understanding, Annie had a total full-on experience of desire to provide sex for David. She has not ever needed him to repeat that or remind her.

And, once their sex life was falling into place more easily, there was more joy and ease between them. And that led to all sorts of freedom, David doing more with all the kids, and Annie feeling so much more supported when she needed to turn her attention to work.

I am not suggesting that sex is the solution to all your problems, but, in this case it was a great starting point. I am sharing this with you to give you an example of things that look to be big issues, and immovable, that people (like me) spent years in therapy with, but with the right tools comes the right leverage. We can actually lift and move things along very quickly.

It is not easy, but it is effective. The work that I am sharing here is not light nor fluff. It will challenge you to your core and shake all your bad behaviors and excuses loose. It is intended to give you back to you first and from there support your life. It will also give you back love in your relationships by transforming them into relational partnerships – if you commit to doing the work.

I use this work every day as I work toward loving relational partnerships in all areas in my life.

If we really look at what is not working, we very soon see that so many little and some big things are starting to fail in the stress of your life and that there are only two possibilities to choose from that will fix this. One is to deconstruct everything and challenge everything detail by detail; the other is to take in the whole big picture of your life and find out how to address it all as One Big Thing. We are going to do the latter. If you have anywhere near all I had going on in my life in yours, this will be a huge relief to you.

This is what has worked for me. Instead of trying to balance your life, I will be inviting you on a journey to transform the culture of your life so that it supports you well and you can have everything you want. The one big thing that we are going to address is your personal culture and, first, the source or foundation of that. These are the two primary components of your love intelligence, or LQ, which we talked about in the last chapter.

Your source is the essence or foundation of who you are choosing to be. Your personal culture is you being the choice you have made; what and who you are saying you are and want to be accountable to be, and who you are proud of being as your life unfolds. This is the aspect of your life that you work toward when we talk about character and values, and yet it is bigger than that. It is who you are choosing to be, what you stand for, what you love, and what moves you. Essentially, it is you. Your source is the choice point. Your personal culture derives from that.

So here we are about to embark on an adventure together. It has a few specific steps to support you, and mainly I will be inviting you on a new adventure of life. Not a change, so to speak, but a transformation in the way you see (possibly) everything. You will be making a choice, one that will impact every area of your life; in a good way.

In this unique paradigm you are being introduced to, these skills follow the structure of sourcing yourself from the oneness field. This is done so that you will have the best opportunity to access your power, choose your personal culture, and ultimately be able to create powerful relational partnerships to fulfill and support your life. Life works with you in alignment with your heart, and with strong partnerships to support you. We are going to address who you are and the state of being that you are in when you are in your life. Then we will take on what you want. These are not "tools," – more appropriately, they should be named "secrets everyone should know."

The results are not finite or easily definable; they will grow and change, and you will too as you use them and as your understanding deepens.

Once we have tackled the source of your life, we will take on your personal culture, what you want and need to live the life of your dreams. First the who you want to be, then the what and how you want to be it.

Together, we will start with a high-level conversation about this. We will embrace a foundational way to create a structure in your life that works across every area of your life; not a piecemeal approach, a whole-life approach. When I discovered that being who I wanted to be was less about following a set of rules or mandates and more about letting myself choose a global solution I could be happy with, that was a huge relief to me.

Many of you who are reading this book certainly have a sense and desire for contribution and recognition of your skills and talents, a family that feels your love and care, an extended family you care about, a world that you care about and are responsible about your relationship to, and a relationship with your husband that includes enjoying your sexual expression. These are some of the components of your personal culture. They also contain your values and the rules you live by – what is important to you, what you love. We will be examining how you define you as your best self after we define your source.

Part 1: What Is the Source of Your Life?

Source: The Basis of a Healthy Personal Culture

The first part of this process is based on the quote from Einstein mentioned before that has influenced me from the moment I first read it over twenty years ago. We are looking for a way to be at ease in our lives, where we can step away from suffering and step into a way of being and seeing that leaves behind the drama and chaos that appears to be inevitable and instead embrace a flow that unfolds gracefully in tune with what we want. Often we think the issue is outside of us with our partner, our children, our community, or our work. I will ask you to consider for a moment that it is very possibly within us, and that it is up to us to find it. The issue might be the way we are looking or what we are looking at that is creating the problem. A consciousness that blames others or puts things outside of ourselves can actually get in the way of the solution. Einstein would have us know that in order to solve our problem, really solve it, we are going to have to radically change something about how we see the world around us.

"No problem can be solved
from the level of consciousness
in which it was created."

– Albert Einstein

Now we will have the chance to explore what this means.

On our way to defining our Personal Culture, we must first choose our Source, or level of consciousness, that Einstein refers to above. This is the crucial decision upon which the rest of the work will rest.

One Foundation: Sourced from Love or Fear

There are two choices as you consider the source or foundation of your personal culture. The choice of the "level of consciousness" that Einstein refers to above; is the source of all your action and is a major factor in the quality of your life. If you have a consciousness that lives in fear, makes trouble, creates problems, and judges others, you will have very different behaviors and outcomes in your life than if you choose a consciousness that is fluid and accepting and loving. Your consciousness is the source of everything within you. It is the one factor that you can change that will affect every area of your life.

The choice is simple; will you choose fear or love? What is normal is to choose fear or to choose love *and* fear and go back and forth, creating a chaotic experience of your life. Sometimes we choose to think well of others and think from love, but often that is a hard choice, an inconvenient choice, and therefore, out of fear or doubt or worry, or desire to dominate or win, we choose fear.

If you choose to be an outlier, choosing love and living into that choice as much as you can is a discipline and a challenge that you will face your whole lifetime. It won't be easy. Fear will come in and derail you, but your commitment to finding your way back to love will make all the difference. And it will be worth it. You will become its student.

This process is one that we used to call "building character." We must choose our foundation or source wisely, otherwise we will be building a 'character' that lacks the necessary component consciousness and values of the life you want to live.

There are no shortcuts on this journey; it is rich and rewarding to choose the source of your personal culture that actually gives you the deepest experience of who you are and will be the source of what you want. I can guarantee that if there is alignment in your source and in your personal culture, there will be ease and alignment in your life.

If you choose to source yourself from loving, you will be open to an expansive life of full expression and possibility.

Stepping into the Field

"Out beyond ideas of right doing and
wrong doing there is a field, I will meet you there...
when two souls lie down in the grass
even the words "each other" make no sense."

– Rumi

The Unified Field; the Consciousness of One; Love and Wholeness.

The most intensely in touch most people get with this field is when they experience falling in love or, often, childbirth. When we fall in love, we are given the gift that was there all along; the love that is in us, that sees the other as the same as us. In this stage, there is no judgment of the other, they are perfect and so are we. This is also the potential state that we can reach in connection with others when we choose to be in the field.

While this all may seem somewhat foreign to you on a day to day basis, you have already resided in this field many times without knowing it. When you feel happy and grateful and loving, creative and alive and full of joy, when you have patience and kindness and integrity, these are all qualities of this field, and therefor denote times that you have been there.

Everything changes for us when we are in this field, everything. We feel safe. Our physiology changes and we are delivered into our parasympathetic nervous system. We are dosed from within with serotonin, dopamine, and oxytocin; the chemistry of love. We give it to ourselves. Our minds open, becoming collaborative and creative. We see beauty and innocence everywhere, our hearts open, and we feel our connection to everything.

When we use the term Love with a capital L, we are focusing our attention on the most powerful and potent force in the Universe. What I am speaking of is a Love Intelligence that lives within us and is being defined by a new framework referred to as LQ. It is beyond personal experience and into an experience of the source of our human capacity to love. In this Love Intelligence, we are paying attention to what is possible when we align with forces for good: when that which is already connected to us connects us deeply to each other. Yes, some would call it God, but that has too many confounding definitions and connotations and too much baggage. Instead, using the term "the Field," gives us the opportunity to acknowledge the sense of wholeness that exists within us and the resonance that it creates around us as well. Acknowledging that there is an organizing power for good that holds us in its field is essential, and I am going to call that power Love.

In this work together, I will use the name The Unified Field for the field in which the power is Love. This concept has its roots in the discoveries of quantum physics. The most important characteristic of this field is that *all is one*; it exists only in the presence of a full joining of us together. We are not merely connected in this field, we are immersed in it as one. Each of us is a hologram of the whole; we each have all the attributes of the whole. None is smaller or less than another. It is mind expanding just trying to wrap your brain around this, but it is worth the effort. Oneness is not a rule we can break or a guideline we can negotiate with. It is the truth of the field. Just as gravity is a truth of this temporal world and is always operating here, oneness is intrinsic in how the unified field operates. When we are in touch with it, it provides us with a sense of power and safety that leads us to our best selves.

If you choose the unified field of oneness as your source, you will be open and available with focus and intention to receive all the gifts of a generous Universe.

Seem a little hard to believe? Or a little too good to be true? Try it on first. Maybe then it will make sense. This is the realm beyond the portal of religion where we can all access the joy of living in "Heaven on Earth." When we can source ourselves from a loving consciousness, we can stay in our bodies and are able to experience the power of the full experience of feeling alive. We are open to our intuition and the guidance that is trying to offer us hints of what feeds our soul. This is where our bodies are calm enough to feel, to soften, and to share with each other. This is the realm of human relationships where we care deeply and feel deeply, with trust and intimacy. It brings us into a connection where we nourish and nurture each other deeply, soul to soul, engaging through our physical human bodies in intimate and sexual partnerships as well.

As long as we cooperate with this truth we can keep our connection alive and create a beautiful life of our dreams; as soon as we get scared, we forget, lose touch, let ourselves judge ourselves or others, or pit ourselves against each other, we step into a realm that is based in fear and instinct. As soon as that happens we enter the other field; the field of duality. Judgment, scarcity, fear, instinct, and separation are always operating as your source in this other field.

The Duality Field; The Field of the Consciousness of Two: Fear, Judgment, Blame, Instinct and Survival

Duality is the field where we don't feel safe; so we are always trying to make that happen; but unfortunately when we are coming from a consciousness of fear and scarcity, we can't. We defeat ourselves as we constantly are working with comparison, competition, and judgment. The questions of right/wrong, good/bad, top dog/underdog, and of course the classic, my God/your God run rampant in this field. Here we are subject to the sympathetic nervous system. The chemistry of that system is adrenalin, and leaves us in a heightened state of agitation and tension when it is not released, leaving lactic acid and uric acid behind and creating the experience of pain in our bodies. It is the field of our human pain and our abandonment as we struggle and strive each day to get everything we 'deserve.' This is the realm that most often resembles the suffering of "Hell on Earth."

Begin to consider, which do you choose? The choosing is important; we will always go back and forth to some degree (perhaps what we call the human experience) because our hardwired limbic system, our amygdala, and reptilian instincts and brains will jump in to save us when there is a perceived threat, large or small. The more we choose oneness, and the more we practice calming and rewiring our brains, the more we will create a space of responsiveness within us. When we can do this, we can move back and forth with agility, eventually having more time in the internal experience of wholeness which brings out our kinder and more loving selves.

This is where we begin:

When things aren't working smoothly in your life, we will look together for the source of the problem. Without judgment we go deep and we look to see the basic assumptions, beliefs, and structures that are holding up the way that life is unfolding for you. I will invite you to accept where you are and analyze that for how it is working, and not. In addition, I will explain to you, show you and give you a sense of how to shift and transform the most basic assumptions of your life to give you the results you are looking for. We will look together for what currently is your source, and what you base your safety in, and then we will offer you an opportunity to look at other possibilities that will give you the most effective ability to live the life of your dreams with grace and peace and joy each day.

While it is hard wired in our brains to come from fear as the result of being based in our instinctual reactivity, we are going to invite you to be at choice in the field of loving as much as possible in order to create a personal culture that works and a life that works. Our lives work when our partnerships are tended to with love and care. And, we can't do this alone.

Part 2: Defining Your Personal Culture – Where Are You Sourced, Who Are You, What Do You Stand For, and What Do You Love?

In this section, I will introduce you to a secret, a key to your life: trying to do everything alone is against the natural order of things. We think we should naturally know how to work together, but actually quite the opposite is true. Instinctually our survival is based on coming together for safety, but when that safety is threatened, we will default surviving alone. We must partner with each other, but most relationships are started and built on instinct and don't have the components to really free both people to work together well. It plays against our fear instinct to do what it takes to relate with vulnerability and authenticity (two key components good partnership) so most of us have little experience in how to do things together effectively. If we turn to our instincts to provide guidance we will fall into the limbic and reptilian system that will usually invite us into the modern-day equivalent of kill or be killed. We hate to admit it. But we might as well.

As we explore the three components of personal culture, we are beginning to discover the basis of healthy relationships which we will call relational partnerships. They are (1) your relationship with the Universe, (2) your relationship with yourself, and (3) your relationship with others. Looking at these three areas will help you set the stage for what you want to create, who you want to be in your life, the person you are proudest of being, all while getting the life you want. You will discover your values and how they show up in your relationships and help define your personal culture, this next level of creation is derived from your source: the core of your love intelligence, or LQ.

Each one of these explorations below will offer you a specific choice point, where you will choose who you want to be. This will go a long way to determining your results in this area. You will have full freedom in the opportunity to choose your way and powerful opportunity to create your results.

After we choose our source, we will explore each of these three areas together, then we will put those results together for a personal culture that you will want to live with in your life. As we explore you will discover what is important to you, and what you stand for, what your values are, what your needs are, and what your dreams are.

You and Life Itself

In the first component part of the process, you need to look at you in relation to your Universe of Life around you. You are the most important component of the personal culture that you are developing. The first orientation will be your relationship with life itself, and how that influences your relationship to the life you choose to have in the world around you. Your relationship with life itself is your relationship to the unseen. The many names for it include, Universal Intelligence, Love, God, the Divine, Higher Power … this will give us a basis from which to start exploring how you want to interact with life.

You and You

The second component of the process is your relationship with you. How do you see yourself in your life? What do you think of yourself, what are your values, the needs and desires that you have? This is a deeply sacred process of inviting you into an awareness of how you hold yourself in relationship to you. These are big questions and once answered can give us leverage to create with. You will be invited into a new way to find yourself, to support yourself in having what it takes to live a happy, joy-filled life that is full of responsibilities, people, and challenges without having to give yourself away to have all that.

You and Others

The third component will show you how to be with, support, and create powerful partnerships with others that will give you the power to leverage all that you are doing in your life and have fulfillment in connection with others. With partnership, with this type of relational partnership, all of that is possible. Your journey will include rich opportunities for growth, love, caring, giving, and receiving. Without partnership, this will be a different journey, you will be faced with different choices. All are valid.

This "You and Others" model is based on a model of partnership as the most fulfilling way to create your life. It is based in alignment with source in the field of loving where all are One. In order to fully access that field, we must create partnerships. It is intrinsic in the flow that we thrive the most in shared space with each other, caring for, and giving and receiving.

In the dualistic field, rather than this, we often get into an instinctual fear-based cutting off of connection, separation, and creating alone. It is not that we never create alone in the partnership model, but when it becomes a way of protecting ourselves from others it limits our vulnerability and our joy. Because of that, the majority of the rest of this book will be focused on leveraging partnerships in all three areas as a route to the greatest levels of satisfaction and ease and to living happily in the life of your dreams.

Partnership is an intrinsic factor for fulfillment in your personal life, your family life, your work life, and your sex life; in fact, it is inherent in life itself. This is far from the popular modern untruth that the people in our lives make our lives harder, turning relationships into jobs of maintenance, management, control, and chaos. You will be able to see and identify that not only is that fallacy not true, but in reality, having many more people in our lives actually makes our lives more free, more joyful, more valuable, more fulfilling, more powerful, and, finally, more at peace.

Your Personal Culture

Finally, in this last chapter of Part 2, after you have chosen your source, and all three of the areas above have been mined for the loves, wants, needs, and desires of your life, you are ready. We will create the actual experience of developing your personal culture.

**"If the idea of partnership with the three components of life (life itself, with yourself, or with others) does not resonate with you, we can work together to find a way to invite the best experience for you that you can create without partnership. We will have a unique exploration and discovery of how this will work for you. This, however, won't be addressed in the scope of this book and is available through private coaching on my website, www.katherinemcclelland.com.

In completing Step One, choosing your Source, and Step Two, examining your values and needs and defining your personal culture, you will complete the first part of this process. You will have what you need to recognize and source yourself and your world. You will have found your way to integrating and defining your personal culture for now, and we will begin the next steps of the journey into Step Three, owning the skills that are necessary as you embark on your journey of partnership. I will refer to these partnerships as relational partnerships in an attempt to distinguish them from relationships based on instinct.

I want to set you up to have the best possible chance to actually realize the life of your dreams. That will take us into our next steps of the LQ system to support you in that.

Part 3: How to Get What You Need from Everyone*

*(Okay well, perhaps not everyone, but everyone who wants to create partnership with you for sure.)

The Four Ingredients for Growth and Sustainability in Relational Partnership: The Love Intelligence Quotient, or LQ, System

Listening, hOnoring, Valuing, and Empowering Ourselves, and Each Other in Relational Partnerships

In this section, I will introduce you in greater depth to the concept of Love Intelligence, or LQ, as coined by Jack Ma (founder of Alibaba Group and self-made billionaire) and to the four essential ingredients of LQ as it pertains to relational partnerships. It is the final link to a love intelligence potential that we all carry within us. and is an essential factor in living our most rewarding and satisfying lives.

As we explore these concepts, you will be learning what it takes to create a system of partnership that creates a culture in which people thrive. In each area, I'll give you resources to make a difference in your partnerships and get the results you want. The overall experience of more giving and receiving, more love, more kindness, more honor and respect, and more freedom will be the same in all areas of your life, the specifics will be different. While it is true that what you want (business, home, husband, kids, friendships, and others) will be specific to those areas, all will bring you more happiness and peace. The following LQ skills will support you well.

The Four Keys to Your Love Intelligence, LQ: The LOVE System of Relational Partnerships

1. *Listening and Speaking: The Possibility of Innocence (Trustworthiness)*

   You will become familiar with the concept of listening and speaking as it pertains to your Love Intelligence and the inevitable sense of connection and power that will result from the assumption of innocence. Trust is a vital component of partnership and will lead to the possibility of vulnerability and authenticity that will develop out of this work. You will see how your past behaviors compare with this and why, for your best life, you will want to create your future behaviors with this in mind.

2. *hOnor: Honor*, Respect, Integrity, Diversity, Kindness, and Authenticity

   You will become familiar with these concepts as they pertain to the sense of connection and goodwill in all types of relational partnerships. You will see the benefit and power of inclusiveness and respect that allows for all types of freedom and creativity to flow from these practices for everyone.

3. *Value: Appreciation, Prizing, Gratitude, and Acknowledgment* You will become familiar with the power of valuing life, yourself, and others. This will inevitably invite a sense of belonging and care amongst people. You will continue to deepen your awareness of partnership as your field of understanding grows. As you do so you will experience a sense of connection, appreciation and gratitude for yourself and your partners even more powerfully.

4. *Empower: Accountability, Guidance, Trust, and Forgiveness* You will be shown the power of the use of very careful accountability shifts through the use of these skills. The responsibility for this type of empowered accountability belongs to both parties and is especially effective with the use of simple guidance, forgiveness and healing that is a part of this process. You will see the opportunity for higher level results in all areas of life.

Part 4: The Possibility of Having It All

And in the end, as we bring you home to yourself, we also bring you into the *one* thing that trips most of us up as we work through this way, or any other way of being a growing human being in this life. It is a big leap to really put your life first and choose to invest in yourSelf, I guarantee that your results, for you, in your life, will be priceless.

Keeping yourSelf present. I will make sure that you are acquainted with the pitfalls that are inevitable as you go through this process. We don't see *all that it takes* to add something as powerful as this to your life. With all of the possibility and change that will naturally come forward, many people will hit the edge of their comfort zone and lose momentum or lose their commitment to themselves when faced with something new. Change, good or bad, triggers our fears and survival instincts, and unless you learn how to establish your presence, keep yourSelf present, heal what is within you that is getting in the way, and keep yourSelf safe, the partnerships you need to create with, will not survive and you will not be able to maintain or sustain the personal culture that you are working so hard to create. You will see the importance of this final skill and the power of solving the problem that losing yourSelf will have on your whole life.

Where we usually falter here, is that we need more support for ourselves than we are willing to ask for. When taking on a transformation, it is necessary for us to invest in ourselves in every area. For me to arrive at this juncture in a happy fulfilling life, I have immersed myself in thirty years of training and development, in coaching and support. I have invested and risked to learn and integrate these tools and concepts into my life, and now I want to bring them to you. I found that it was integral to my success to invest my time, my money, and my heart if I really wanted to make a difference in my life. I was challenged to stand on the shoulders of those who taught me by adapting and integrating my learning into my own creation. I gave all these tools to myself first, that is how I knew what I wanted to give you. This system works, not because of you, or me, because of a mutual commitment to the key components of Love Intelligence. Because I have honed what I have learned, it will not take thirty years for you to create the transformation that you want in your life. I have created something new for you that is faster and more readily available. It will require a fierce commitment from you. If you do choose to invest in yourself, your life will pay you back in more ways than you can even dream.

I will share one avenue of finding a powerful space for yourSelf to shine from within you as we explore the world of Raw Naked Beauty, a process for women to reclaim their radiance and beauty from the inside and get immediate results in confidence, alignment, and empowerment for themselves, their lives, and relationships.

Preparation and Integration: You will be able to see how this Love Intelligence framework will enhance your life. You will be able to choose your source to create the foundation for your personal culture. In addition, once you decide on the components of your specific personal culture, you will be able to use the LOVE key ingredients of that system to create the relational partnerships that support you having the life you want. These partnerships are the key to having what you need to support your happiness and enjoyment in having it all: work, family, and love. And you will know you can do this on your own, and, if you want a route that will be faster, easier, and more likely to be successful, I am available to coach you in the understanding and transformation that is possible in the integration of the work presented in this book. Thank you for your interest in my book I have left my heart print on these pages in my desire to share these thoughts and my desire for you to live every day in the life of your dreams. Please feel free to contact me through my website for questions or follow up coaching. I will be happy to share more with you.

LQ: Love Intelligence:
Part 2–

Defining Your Personal Culture –

Where Are you Sourced, Who Are You, What Do You Stand for, and What Do You Love?

As we begin this journey together, employing these "ways of being" below will bring you the greatest success on our journey together. In choosing to embody these qualities, you will be bringing your whole self to the task of living your dream life.

Being your whole self is your part of our journey. So before you jump all the way in, look at this list below and check the ones you know you can embody right now. Your willingness to use and strengthen the ones you already know, and to embrace, and learn those you aren't familiar with, will give you the best chance to mine the material in this book to live the life of your dreams.

Ways of being your whole self, or who you are being as you do what you do:

- Be open to learn
- Be ready to grow
- Be kind
- Be helpful
- Be YourSelf
- Live from your heart
- Be ready to bleed
- Be ready to let go
- Be ready
- Be present
- Be authentic (tell the truth about what you think, who you are, and what you want)
- Be loving
- Be magical
- Be willing to be healed.
- Be willing to be happy
- Never ever guess why something is happening
- Drop the story and live into the miracle

- Assume innocence of All in every situation
- Know that you are Loved
- Be in Love
- Love and care for You First
- Love and care for All as You

Be ready to fail, to fall, and to bleed but just don't give up. Your ego, the part of you that gets scared and that separates you and wants you to be perfect? It won't like this at all.

This process is not for your ego, it is for you and will give You back to you.

"You do not belong to you. You belong to the Universe.
The significance of you will remain forever obscure to you,
but you may assume you are fulfilling your significance
if you apply yourself to converting all you experience to
highest advantage to others.
Make the world work, for 100% of humanity, in the shortest
possible time, through spontaneous cooperation, without
ecological offense or the disadvantage of anyone."
– Buckminster Fuller

Chapter 4 reflecting on and choosing

CHAPTER 4

Reflecting on and Choosing Your Source

Two Fields, One Choice

Here's a hard truth: No matter what you are thinking about how all the people in your life are not pulling their weight, not doing their part, leaving things to you to handle, no matter what you are thinking about how alone you are and how this always happens, no matter what you are thinking about how you have to demand and push and manipulate to get others to help.... You are wrong.

It is not happening to you. It is happening because of you. Your blind spots are creating your reality.

Sensing that you might have just thrown this "stupid book" across the room now, I will hope that you will pick it back up.

Hopefully, it will help if I tell you that even though it is because of you, even though it is your responsibility to change it, that's actually the good news.

And if that doesn't make sense to you yet, I will spell it out here; since it is yours, we can correct it. The demise of your life is not inevitable. It will be a choice. It will be your choice. You will not be able to control the outcomes, but you will be able to choose who you want to be, who you are being in every moment. Things will change, but that does not have to result in destruction. Who you are being, in each moment, is what will change your life. I am here to offer you the choice about that. This chapter will clearly delineate how that is so.

We are going to go on a journey together, a deep dive into what is behind the you that shows up in the world each day. You will see as we travel together that as you are able to see what is behind your upset, overwhelm, and, possibly, the sense of futility in your life, there is essentially a simple choice that will give you back – or for the first time – what you really want.

We have a tendency to think that life is random and just happens to us. That everything comes together for some people, or falls apart for some. We don't realize that without knowing it, we set ourselves up to win or fail. I'd like to set you up to win.

Another idea that seems to run us is that if we just push hard enough for a little bit longer, the results we want will magically appear. What you might notice is that that is not what happens at all. Yes, we might get a break, go on vacation, or make it through a crisis, but either you take the thing that is not working on vacation with you, or it is waiting for your return. In the case of a crisis handled, another one is right around the corner. The fact that things feel out of control is because they are. There is something missing in your underlying structure and, it is not more control. And we are going to explore that and have you return that to yourself.

As we look at the basic structure underneath the feelings of overwhelm, anxiety, and frustration, we see that the deeper source of these experiences is all the same. And the good news is, we can change that. The tricky part is that it is going to require some basic changes in your structure if your structure is not working.

My client Kathy was very frustrated in her life. She felt like just when she would get on top of things, something would go wrong and she would have a mess on her hands. When she came to me to work on this, she felt really distraught. She felt like she did not get life and how to do it. She was hoping that I could offer her something like a rulebook – how to get life right. What the steps were. I really understood how she was feeling and would have loved to have provided that for her. But, of course, there is no rulebook, unless you just pick someone else's and live by that. I didn't recommend that to her, nor will I to you. And, with the very same process that we will be exploring here, Kathy was able to choose her source and structure, define her life, make some pivotal choices that lead to transformation in the basis of her life, and get back to creating what she wanted in her life.

That's what I want for you.

What we will be looking at and embracing in this chapter is developing a sense of your source. You may not even know there is a source of you but there is. It is invisible to most of us. Your source is behind everything you do, it is the basis for your structure of beliefs, and a sense of safety or fear that directs you. This is the source of what you will come to know as your personal culture.

Your source is the basis of you, the you that goes everywhere with you. The one that supports you or tears you down. The one that takes you out of the fight or gets you in it. The one who gives you back to your peace. Or the one that destroys everything and everyone around you. That One. Whichever one it is. It is the you you are choosing, the you you are being. And, once you identify it, you can choose what you want.

There are only two choices of your Source. What runs in the background of your life is going to run your life. The first choice is based in survival and fear (which calls on our older brain systems that are hard-wired on high alert to you,) and its only capacities are reactive and will put us into adversarial situations constantly defending, demanding, manipulating and assaulting for what we want. The second choice is based in the consciousness of expansion, or what we will also refer to as your Love Intelligence. It is wired into the 'newer' brain systems and is wired to calm you and help you see the bigger picture. This is the system that invites us to higher thinking, to altruism, and to being the people we are proud to be. This part of you is your higher self.

Whichever one is running in the background, is running your life. One of our big questions is are you choosing for you or is your brain choosing for you?

All of us, without choosing, vacillate between these two sources of life constantly. When we are settled and calm with our needs met, we are much more able to be in our source of expansion and love intelligence, our Self. When we are at all rushed, hungry, angry, or trying to juggle too many things, we will inevitably push ourselves into our survival system.

The difference is vast. They are not shades of the same thing, they are two totally different systems with vastly differing results for your life. Your survival is always there and waiting to take over when it thinks you are not getting it right. It is your fail safe. It's good to have in case you are being attacked by a lion or are bleeding out, just not good to have in charge in your day-to-day life.

Our hidden survival selves, from a mind of fear, live in a world characterized by judgment, separation, attack, assault, demand, lying, cheating, and manipulating for the results we think we want or need. We are not "bad people," our motivating mind has us on hyper drive to get what we think we need to survive. That is its only job, the real bottom line.

When the source of our personal culture is based in survival or fear, we have a life that can feel hard and lonely. The more we relate to others from behind a veil of that fear, the more we hide our truth, the more we pretend we're okay when we're not, the further and further we get from our truest selves, our intuition, our hearts and from each other, and the more pain we have.

Our truest or essence Self lives in a field of love. This higher Self lives in a field that is characterized by a permeating sense of safety, joy, expansion, potency, and power. What is given is also received, what is seen in you is seen in the other, what is good in you is good in the other. For our truest selves, the ends never justify the means that aren't aligned. Everything is held in a coherent field where everything is One. How we treat each other is simply how we treat ourselves. There is no difference.

Both of these systems work in alignment within themselves. If we fight we get fighting, if we love we get loving, if we are afraid we get more afraid, when we are free we get more free.

From our fearful or instinctual selves, we relate to the world and ourselves from a distance with scarcity, worry, doubt, suspicion, control, dominance, and cynicism. When we choose that, we choose that world.

This calls you into your sympathetic nervous system. This is its job. Its job is survival. It has no conscience, no ability to reason. It is only interested in what is best for your survival in any moment. It does not value anything but your physical life. At all costs.

It keeps you on high alert for danger. It looks for trouble and it squelches it.

It has no concept of morality within you, the intrinsic sense of what is right for you. It only knows survival separation, and judgment of others, it's all instinct.

This system of duality or instinct is based in your limbic system, in your amygdala. It is hard-wired into your brain. It is an old system and fueled by adrenalin it only gives you four reactions that you can employ: *fight, flight, freeze, faint*. That's it. That's all we have to use in that system. And it moves in and takes over lightning fast.

There is nothing else that moves faster. You are at its mercy. Until you take charge.

The more time we spend here, the more we are filled with this chemistry, and the more we make up supporting stories of why we should be afraid. The more afraid we are, the more afraid we get. We, our truest selves, get lost. We sacrifice our humanity and honor and dignity. We go into hiding. We become predator, we become prey. And that's all we've got. An endless game of "who will die today so I can be safe."

Alternately, when we choose to move away from fear, and employ a practice to do so, for instance to breathe and move our bodies and our minds out of our fear, we can access our parasympathetic nervous system, and we have more freedom. This is our rest and restore system, this system lets us access the whole of who we are. This system is governed by the chemistry of serotonin, oxytocin, and dopamine. This is love. This is the system that you are bathed in when all is right in your world. It is your healing system within your own body. It is complex, but for now, all we need to know is that as we step into this choice our world changes. Immediately.

What if you could choose to step into this system? A system that has within it all possibilities inherent in the teachings of the mystical teachers, peace, passion, and expansion but is not religious? A system that we also have within us where we are cared for and protected, a system where creativity, compassion, love, and joy, are the foundational experiences of those who choose this source of their personal culture.

For many of us, once we know this, we would just think "Okay, well then I'll choose. I choose my highest Self, my parasympathetic system, and I choose all those attributes that go along with it." And that would be great if it were that simple.

The issue within us is always our safety. If we feel safe, loved, and cared for and with our basic needs met, finding our way to our source of consciousness, our expanded brain that lives in a field of loving, is possible. On the other hand, whenever we sense a threat of any kind, we trigger into survival and give up our higher self and our humanity very quickly. Kill or be killed is the law of this land.

Since our safety is everything to us, it controls how we operate. If your strategy for safety is to find your safety outside of you, through trying to control others, people, places, things, or money, you are always at the mercy of something changing. When things change, as they do, someone you count of steps away from you, you lose your job or your home, someone you love dies, or for any other reason, your sense of control that you have outsourced, is revealed as not real. When you source yourself outside yourself you trigger your amygdala every time something goes wrong. If anything changes, you might die. In this system, you are alone, you think you are better off alone, so you act alone. In our physiology, we human beings are such a vulnerable species; we are hard wired to work together. If you are working alone, you have cut yourself off from a deeper sense of your own natural intelligence and information that will help you make good decisions and keep you safe. Even if you don't think you see it that way, your brain will eventually make you a liar by showing you that you do. If we are safe because of our people and things, we are not really safe because inevitably things will change.

If, on the other hand, you look within and find your source of safety within you, you will be more stable and resilient, not so vulnerable to changes in your life. We all have had moments of gut feelings, "knowing something" that has helped us in knowing what to choose or do. We need the access to this information. If we don't have it, as we don't when we are in our survival brain, we will not have all that we need to keep ourselves alive and aware. If you are willing to begin to experiment with trusting that the Universe might have your back, that there is a net that will catch you, that your innocent acceptance of your love intelligence will allow you to see and hear and use information that can't come to you in a closed system, then you will see different results. When you are in the system of peace and calm, everything is available to guide you. If you are willing to take heart, to be courageous, you will begin to see that you are not alone, and, that we do better together. It is you and the Universe together, it is not you alone that works. It is you and life, you and your divine connection, you and infinite intelligence. The Universe is not chaotic, it is based in good, and your love intelligence is in you, it is here for you.

It can be a challenge to learn this because we must somehow take a leap of faith and choose to trust first, to try it out, and then we will get the results. This is not for the faint of heart but it will give you the freedom and joy and the life you want.

In my story, my triggers were big and had me living in a sense of survival most of the time, something I was unaware of for most of my life. For some of you, your story might be similar so you will recognize the experience, but it is not necessary to have a big story to switch to the survival brain. Something as simple as seeing your husband look at another woman, changing jobs, or your child getting sick, can trigger us easily. So if you don't have a big story, all you need are the regular influences in daily life, a bad night's sleep, no breakfast, and children, bosses, work, clients, husbands, and life demands can all switch our brains to survival mode and leave our deeper selves banished outside our awareness, shivering in the rain. Let's come in out of the storm and discover this place of safety, stability, and peace together.

The Beginning of the Journey of Understanding Alignment with Source

In order to really explain this journey, I am once again going to take you into my life to explain how I discovered this paradigm and ultimately my alignment with Source. It grew out of my need to feel safe in my very unsafe world. I want to assure you before we go in, that while it was very intense, I am fine. I have found what I need to heal and this was the journey home to myself.

Your journey will likely not be as dramatic, and I am only telling you this so that you can see how I got to my understanding, how it came to be that, finally overwhelmed by fear, I had to source my own safety. That gave me the tools to help others.

I began my journey to understanding this when, as an underage patron in a bar in Washington DC, I was confronted with this inscription on the bathroom wall. I was sixteen and it has never left me.

> *"fighting for peace is like screwing for virginity"*
> – bathroom wall, Gallagher's pub, Washington DC

As a sixteen-year-old savvy beyond my years, having grown up overseas in a place where violence was almost always breaking through into our lives, or about to, I knew and understood how absolutely insane it is to fight for peace. And, as for the second part, there were plenty who had been trying to relieve me of my virginity for years – I could tell all that groping and touching was not for my virginity. From this quote, in an instant, what I really got was that you can't be doing two opposing things at the same time. You can't be fighting for peace or hurting each other for love.

You can't be living in your brain of fear and enjoying a life of peace.

I grew up in a world of violence and danger. My father was an American diplomat stationed in the Middle East. My birth country was Saudi Arabia, then we were off to Lebanon, Iraq, Iran when the Shah was in power for safety, and then on to Kuwait and Egypt. Most of my childhood was spent behind one wall or another guarded by machine gun-toting guards with varying degrees of training – supposedly this was for my safety. But of course, I did not feel safe.

The threats were real and everywhere. And so, when the tanks rolled down the streets and the bombs started to drop out of the sky, when the guard put a machine gun to my head, when twenty-four of them met me at the door demanding entry, I already knew I would never be safe in that world.

The danger in my early years was both in and outside of my home. Unfortunately, some of my biggest influences involved sexual trespasses (#metoo) moments with those in whose care I had been entrusted but who were not a reliable source of safety for me. Locked doors, friendship, honorable people, none of them provided the safety that was promised for me.

Since that time, I had been searching for and yearning for a world I could be safe and happy in. I knew there must be a different answer. At that point, I was so afraid, and I was choosing to get smaller and smaller in my world. I built the big walls within that I lived behind as a child. And one day I realized, it was not only keeping others out, it was restricting my freedom and keeping me hidden within. As that was happening, I couldn't hear the voices within that were trying to give me access to myself and my safety. I was still looking outside me for a place, a person, or something I could carry that would ensure my safety and peace.

And I was struggling and not present in my life. I was so busy hiding that I put everything inside, zipped it up and went about my life trying to figure life out; to do it right, to figure out rules to live by.

Your life might not have looked like mine in specific, but in life, it seems to be the way, that we are all susceptible to this same place, the trespasses that you have endured, the fears that you have internalized, even just the striving for attention may have left you in a place where some of this struggling feels familiar.

Some part of me thought this was just me. But as I studied and lived and was finding my way, I started to realize that our brains trigger very easily and you don't need to have anything but an experience where you feel somehow hurt or threatened to know the reality of what it feels like to live in fear in your mind.

This was the beginning of my journey to seeing and understanding the two sources that create the two types of personal culture. At that time, I looked around the world and I began to see that my world and the personal cultures of everyone around me involved duality; a right and wrong, good and bad, fear scarcity and separation mentality. In that world, I could be your friend one day and your enemy the next. We were all choosing from a sense of judging each other from fear, who was right and wrong, good and bad. It included the worlds of all the religions I had been exposed to.

I knew there was a better way.

When I got to the teachings of Gandhi I heard the saying "an eye for an eye makes the whole world blind." I knew I had found one of my teachers. I saw that if I retaliated then the other would just feel justified retaliating against me. This was a no-win situation. I understood that it couldn't be both ways. If I wanted love and oneness, then I had to choose love and oneness and kindness and care of as the source of personal culture. In Gandhi's culture, in this the world that he created, every person was respected. While behavior that was outside of loving, care, and honor for the other was not tolerated and, the "crime/behavior," disallowed, the person remained intact and cared for with respect and honor. I knew that a source that respected and honored all was the only source that would ever provide safety or care unconditionally. It is the only way it can be, and the only one that I could ever trust.

Your source is your choice. It is the ultimate choice. From this source of oneness, there is nothing outside of love. When you adopt a source like this, you give yourself to your most expansive possibilities, the most powerful opportunities of life. This is a very healthy system with complete wholeness.

Once I knew that my source was love, I began looking for a personal belief system I could live with and a personal culture I could live within, and dedicated my life to finding it. I looked everywhere, studied many cultures, religions, and philosophies, all in an effort to find the one that would practice what I wanted to hear. Peace and love were my highest values. I looked everywhere.

I began to find them, but in many places, even when people were kind and loving within a community, I was still confronted with the fact that anyone outside of the specific community I was studying in was separated out, vilified, judged, and set apart as unclean/bad/crazy or just plain wrong.

In this kind of thinking, the consciousness of love cannot exist. When something is placed outside the field, it puts the whole field out of integrity. We are back to choosing sides and fighting for peace.

Because all of our systems are run by people who have instincts of right and wrong, the religious path, political systems, our society, could not keep themselves from making others wrong, so then, there was no peace. It is possible to disagree without vilifying the other, but that is not how most people do it.

Perhaps because of my early experiences, I was very sensitive to separating out people, vilifying them, and making them wrong. I had been unfairly separated out and vilified for being American, for being blond, for being white, for being a girl to name a few. And, I had known and been cared for (and not) by people from many cultures, ways of life, and religions. I was clear that culture/color/religion/gender were not the demarcations of safety and love; it was the consciousness of the individual person that made all the difference about whether I was safe with them or not. If they were sourced from love I was safe; if they were sourced from fear, there was a good chance I was not safe. When that was the case, in many ways in those moments, they were not themselves. They were operating out of a system that has no conscience, and thinks it is fighting for its survival.

As I searched in my life, I went through two marriages, and many challenges. My family relationships always seemed in a shambles. I hated the chaos and the upset and yet I participated. My nervous system was on high alert, I was undone. I could not settle in unless I did a lot of meditation to calm myself, but I had no more time. The harder I worked, the more kids I had, the more I had what I wanted, the more I tried to do the right thing, the worse it got. Others judged me, I judged myself, I judged them. I couldn't feel all the love that I had started my marriage with. I knew I was failing everyone, even with the best of understanding and intentions.

I was failing. I was stuck behind my wall of fear. My wall of fear did not always feel like fear. It felt like anger, and contempt and judgment of others, but it was, in the end, based in fear.

And then I began to read more spiritual texts. *A Course in Miracles*, the mystical traditions of Christianity, *The Dead Sea Scrolls*, the Sufi traditions, the Kabbalah, the teachings of Yogananda. As I attended school for spiritual psychology, I started to find those who were searching for the same ideals, the same peace, and I started to find the source of a personal culture I could live with. Finally, in the teaching of the school, I found those who believed in a source that was beyond right and wrong, one that invited me into a wholeness with the rest of life. A culture where behavior could be okay or not okay, but one where no one was dishonored even if they were not allowed to continue the behavior. It was up to the group to sort out the plan for things to be made right, but in the ideal, no person was shamed and made wrong.

I saw that this culture based in love was not religious, and eventually as I started to explore working within the systems of the human body, I saw that in many ways it wasn't only spiritual either. Choosing a world of peace and love and kindness and creativity is a choice of awareness and understanding, but those choices are not available in a body and mind based in and influenced by fear.

As I began to study this more in depth, I came across the way that this is all reflected in our bodies, reflecting the choices we have in the realms of the mind and the spirit as well. There are simply two sets of choices in every area as we define our source.

Based in our bodies, we can see how we are essentially a two-source world, and how we are choosing from that. No matter what you believe, no matter what is important to you, or what you want or need, you only have two source choices. Either you choose a culture that is sourced from duality and results in personal cultures based in fear, separation and judgment, scarcity, and anxiety, or you find your way to a culture sourced in oneness, which results in personal cultures based in love, honor, and respect, abundance and gratitude.

Your source is not personal. It's a choice. This is your freedom … *or* not. The difference in your life is radical and all-encompassing. It becomes personal, in your personal culture when you add your flavor, your beauty, your particular humanity to it. People who have embodied the choice to be sourced in love and worked over time to find their way within it include Gandhi, MLK, the Dalai Lama. These people each made it personal to them as they added and embodied their own specific and different religious background, each of them found it integral to their work in very different ways. Each one of these people worked every day to find the way to be as loving as they can be while still maintaining a sense of behavioral integrity. If the action wasn't loving, it wasn't okay. Religion is just one portal, it is not a necessary ingredient to this work.

While I am not as accomplished or as consistent as these world leaders, this is the work that I do each day. This is challenging work, but the benefits are powerful and your life will blossom from this place. This is a simple system with a simple choice to make, but it is not easy.

As I came to understand this more and more, I was beginning to see how my world was affected by my choice of source in love and consciousness. When I could choose a consciousness of oneness, I could choose to live in peace and safety and freedom. I was safe and others were safe around me. When I chose from duality, I chose a world of fear and pain and very doubtful outward protection, certain unsafety, and it was a world of fear and judgment, it was that for me and that for others around me too.

I began to see and experience the unspoken reality that each world will give you what you invest. And, as hard as it is to believe, each will give you back exactly what you believe. It is not magic. What you believe sets your destiny.

The first choice is your source. Will you choose love or fear?

If you choose as your source, a field that has within it the consciousness of oneness and loving, you get abundance, joy, grace, partnership, kindness, compassion, and peace. No matter the specifics of your personal culture, you will have this in common with everyone who is sourced from love. You can want different things, choose different lifestyles, earn more or less money than others, those are all choices of your personal culture, but if your source remains the same you can live with each other.

Sourced in love you become uniquely you, you create your own personal culture. You can choose to have a big job, a couple of kids, a lot of help, a gorgeous home, a husband you can't keep your hands off of, and an interest in interacting with the world on a large scale, and someone else can choose to have a stay-at-home life with lots of kids, no husband, homeschooling, raising their own garden, and being together every day, and it doesn't matter – as long as you are sourced in love, it is your world, you get to have it your way.

This is one of the keys to thriving in your very full life. If you allow yourself to choose this expanded field, you will learn to flow in your connection with source, and you will be able to make decisions easily using your own inner guidance system, things become clearer and simpler, you are open and your partnerships easily support you.

When you are settled in your system, you will have access to alternate sources of information, intuition, synchronicity, and support.

If you choose a field that has within it the consciousness of duality and fear, you will often feel the need to protect yourself, your lifestyle, and your choices so you get scarcity, survival, instinct, and against-ness and no help from your 'friends.'

What will you choose?

When did *love* become a four-letter word?

When did we decide that to be led by our love intelligence with honor and respect that we are naïve or simple or not savvy enough? When did we decide that to be against something or someone was more powerful than to be for something or someone? When did we decide that we know more than all of the wisdom of the ages?

When we got scared. When we were taught to be fearful and wary, not to trust but instead, to try to control everything. That's when we lost our contact with the ancient knowing of the truth of the power of our loving consciousness, our love intelligence.

Do you feel like you are living in a world where you have no choice, where you are forced by instinct into duality by our brain? On top one moment, on the bottom the next. Even when you think you will be safe and have made the choice of being wary and closed, distant, and fearful to ensure your safety, there is no real safety in the world of fear. This world is full of suspicion, cynicism, anger, frustration, and danger to all. In fact, the saying "there is no honor among thieves." speaks to this point. If you are making others right or wrong, in effect stealing their humanity, they will for the most part give you the same in return. You only see what you see and you only get what you give.

If you choose this world of instinct, even if you barricade yourself with your people behind your guns and walls, when there are only two of you left, you will choose yourself every time. It is instinct. It is survival. I've seen it. Maybe you have too.

Or will you decide to live in a world where everything is held in a field of love and respect, honor and compassion? As you look you can begin to see the alternate source of consciousness or love. You can begin to see that a world based in oneness and love and peace could be a more practical world. Love intelligence works. People care for each other, listen to each other, share with each other, the world, and the planet. People are happy, caring, and successful, they are honorable and kind, compassionate, and free of fear.

We will begin to explore this culture and see how relationships become partnerships within a culture of acceptance and compassion. We will see how the highest humanity has to offer is called forward in personal cultures sourced from love.

And the lowest instinct-based behavior is called forth in personal cultures sourced from fear. From fear, we inherit scarcity, manipulation, anything that puts us on top without care for others. Even in our alliances we remain adversaries, knowing that if push comes to shove, we will push them under the bus.

It also shows up in smaller ways. Any time we get scared. Angry, upset, hurt, worried, it gives us a small world determined to take everything out that threatens it. And in the process it takes us, who we really are, out.

It is from here that we threaten our partnerships. We assault those we love the most. We are judgmental with those we love the most. We vilify those who are like us but who stray even a little, and those who are not like us at all.

How on earth can we be "in love" when we have a system like this operating within us as our source and a personal culture that defines us by being against bad things?

As we look at this, not from a place of judgment but of pragmatism, what really makes the most sense? Are you willing to see that in this source of fear, and a personal culture based in fear, worry, doubt, and judgment, that you are part of the problem, and are creating most of the pain in your own life? Are you willing to let go of your self-righteousness and be happy?

Should we choose living in fear so we are to be ruled by our ancient nervous system?

Or do we choose to find our way into the power of your love intelligence, opening the parasympathetic system and all the treasures that are given to us from there? This seems like a naturally good choice. And it is, and, the tricky part is, even when you are bought in, you can be derailed by the mighty amygdala in a split second.

Let's say, you are bought in. You love the idea of a system that is based in love and kindness, honor and respect. And then something happens – your husband calls, the kids are sick, and he doesn't have the number to call the vet to keep the dog one more night. And you start to lose it. "Can't he just handle anything?"

Don't say that.

Instead, squeak out: "I'll call you back as soon as I can" and hang up the phone.

Getting back to our hearts when we are captured by our survival instincts is a very very challenging journey; the whole world looks dangerous and adversarial. It looks like you have to control everything, you can't trust anybody. Your heart may be racing with your worries, your eyes darting around, your thoughts bouncing to and fro, and you feel emotional and out of control. These are warning signs that you are being controlled by your amygdala and are not *you*. At this juncture, you are pure instinct. You are tense. And your body is looking for a way to resolve it. The ways that you are thinking of are probably not going to help. They make things worse, especially if there is another human involved. You may harm them or yourself in your effort to survive.

This is where we must find our way home.

Practical Steps to Release the Grip of Adrenalin, Fear, and Survival

Instead of losing it:

First: Breathe. Breathe. Breathe. At least three full deep breaths. All the way down into your belly. At least three more. Breathe. And again. Not silly. Important.

You are attempting to get yourSelf back as you re-align your nervous system. If you are like most busy people, you get caught in the fight/flight/freeze/faint system trying to manage too many things and we can't move into any other reality while it has a grip on us. Breathe.

Second: Move your body. Move it any way you can. Move. Move. Wiggle, or better yet, go outside and go for a walk. Just close your office door and move. If you can yell somewhere safe, do it.

You are still working on your nervous system.

Third: Say something that is true. It is Tuesday. I am a woman. My dog's name is Charlie. I feel angry. I feel hurt, sad, bad whatever. *Do not add the because*, just say what is actually happening right now. Say something that is true.

Do not tell the story to yourself ("because" or…). Whatever it is. If you want to analyze your needs, I will go over that in the next chapter. But for now, do not tell the story again. It is probably not true. It usually starts with things like "He never…" "I always …" "the kids are …" "OMG the dog is driving me…." Don't share the story. Don't listen.

Fourth: Again, tell the truth. Something like: "I am hungry. I have not taken good care of myself today. I have nothing to give right now. I need to get some food and sit down for a minute."

You are still working on your nervous system. And you may be able to sense a loosening of the sensations inside your body. If so, you are headed in the right direction. Keep going if yes or no.

Wash, rinse, repeat. Breathe. Move your body. Tell the truth.

This is the place where Body Intelligence and Love Intelligence meet. In a nod to Kathlyn Hendricks and her BQ work, starting in the body can often give us access to all our other faculties. When we are triggered, working in your body to regulate your nervous system is a great place to start. Then you can take your next steps.

When your system calms down, call him back, handle the immediate need with patience and understanding, and read the rest of the book ASAP.

And now, now that you are calm again, notice *who* you can *be*. Is your mind clear? Do you sense that there are more possibilities than you could think of before?

Can you feel your loving? Do you have a sense of you being right there and present?

That's good. Now. From this place, you can ask difficult questions of yourself and can listen to the answers. This is how you change your results.

I invite you into an inventory of your life.

You are brave to look. You are looking because you will then know how to move forward. You must only do this when you are calm and rested and can support yourself.

Who have you been being in your life? Are you proud of her? Does she listen well and speak kindly to others?

Do you love her or judge her and do you pick on her mercilessly? Is she ever good enough for you?

When are you kind to yourself? Do you want more of that?

What kind of personal culture have you cultivated? Where is it full of judgment and drama, upset and blame? Do you feel the tension in you in these times?

Where do you share kindness? Would you like more love and kindness from yourself?

Which field is your personal culture sourced in? Both? When do you find yourself tense and disconnected throughout your day?

When are you in charge, and responsive and responsible, present and available to yourself?

When are you at the effect of the world around you, letting *the world or others* choose your attention? When do you let your emotions fly off at others? Do you want to be more in charge of that?

Are you operating in a world full of unexpressed and unfulfilled needs?

When do you feel the flow of your energy and goodwill toward others? What happens to time in those different realities?

What parts of your life are full of peace and kindness and partnerships that are supporting the life you are wanting to create?

Look closely – this is pivotal for your life.

Where are you now? Where have you been?

Can you see the moments you have been sourced in fear? And when you are sourced in love?

Can you begin to discern the difference?

What do you want? What do you choose?

I love you. You got this.

CHAPTER 5

Developing Your Relationship with Life through Source

In this chapter, we will discuss the first of the three components of your personal culture. This first component is your relationship with life, from the source that you have chosen. We are going to discuss creating your own personal culture of honor, respect, and care for all of life. The personal culture that gives you back to you. We will be discussing source again to some degree and asking you to begin to choose how you want to interact with life and the components of your personal culture that will support you.

There is a myth that people have been selling for years now, that we can pull our lives apart piece by piece and put them back together and somehow get them more balanced and that that will solve our problems. I'm calling the game on that. I have tried it. In my marriage, in my work/love/family life. My clients have tried it before they came to me. It has resulted in high expectations and high disaster as over and over we try to find how to have everything we want in our lives, every day, without being sourced in ourselves. I know you may not know what that means. You will very soon.

One day I finally knew. There is just no way to balance life enough so it works everyday.

So I began looking for another answer. And I found the one I will be teaching you. The answer falls to the part of the spectrum of life that is called "getting present" and "quiet." It is about taking a deep breath first, relaxing into what is truly happening now, and then finding our answers in an ongoing inquiry of what is motivating you, what you love, what you really need, what you need from others, and how you can truly care for yourself.

Instead of trying to control and anticipate every outcome and set everything right by knowing everything, what to do and how to do it, being perfect and in charge, and on top of every detail, which is how we act when we are in fear, in the system of the consciousness of oneness, in our love intelligence, we have a very different experience. In the love field, you step into openness, trust, and to a life that flows from your source. Through the skills that you will practice in this chapter you will begin to listen and hear the guidance that is all around you. You become attuned to impulses and niggles, nudges, and synchronicities and all the ways your intuition and connectedness speaks to you. You learn to trust as you begin to listen to what calls your attention. Instead of having to pay attention to everything all the time, you define your personal culture and that defines what you care about the most. In time, your system will alert you, without you having to keep track of everything when something is amiss or needs your attention.

I can see how this all might sound a bit unusual, or out of touch with your day-to-day life, but, despite the fact that it is based in a spiritual system, it is down to earth in its application. It will give you the daily life you want, a sense of calm and peace, and love and kindness. This works if you do the work.

While I was still attempting to "balance my life," I was a minister who could love deeply all of the people I saw every day, but, when I went home with nothing left to give, my people, my heart, my closest family suffered. I found this way in order to find my way home within and to be who I wanted to be all day each day.

The whole point of this book is to teach you how to live a life where you are in love every day, how to exchange your upset, anger, fear, sadness, and self-judgment for love and delight, and how to bring the sense of joy, peace, happiness, self-honoring, and creativity into your life every day. And, how to do all that while you live a real life, with real people, real children, and real needs of your own. Heaven on Earth, I say.

When Susan was young, she had a real sense of the path that she wanted to walk. She was going to be successful and powerful in her business. She was going to have a couple kids, a great husband, and a life that worked.

As the reality of that started to settle in, with each passing year, things just weren't going well.

On the outside, it looked okay, but she was beginning to have a sense of being alone on the inside. It felt to Susan like she was working harder but never catching up. And she felt like she just didn't know how to get it right.

She was starting to feel a sense of loss every day. Every day she went to work, she was missing something important at home, and every evening she was feeling like she was distant and distracted from her family because of something she had to leave at work.

She could hardly muster the enjoyment of her family and life just felt like one big chore. And she kept having this niggling pain inside.

What is that? She kept thinking it would go away.

And it didn't. Instead it started to develop into a full-blown sense of dread. Every day, no matter what she was doing, she was not satisfied.

She was beginning to wonder what was wrong with her. Everyone else at work seemed to be handling everything so well, but she could barely keep her head above water. She was sinking and so was her heart and her life. Drowning, actually, is what she said.

As we began to work together, she realized that she had not slowed down in years to look and to find what was in her world and what she wanted. She was running her life based on the expectations of "what everybody else wanted and was doing" and not on what she really wanted to do.

She inevitably sensed that she had no idea how to create a life where she felt good. She just assumed it would fall into place. But it hadn't. In fact it was getting worse. She had no idea what she needed in order to create a life that could fall into place according to her desires, and she had no idea how to get her needs met once she found them.

She was experiencing a lot of resentment in her marriage, leading her to be distant and accommodating but leaving her cold and disconnected. Sex was a chore that she knew she had to fulfill in order to stay married. And she wanted that.

And there was more. Once having seen this, it was obvious that there were many areas to work on and many places she could start.

We could have gone to the many places in her life where she was feeling challenges, frustrations, and out of alignment, but instead, we started with the foundation. Who she was being each day. Where she was sourced and what life or personal culture did she want to choose from there?

This led to a great transformation, with less effort than you might imagine. We were able to pull some ideas and assumptions out by the roots and begin to help her find her source, her true heart's desire, to define the woman she would be proud of being, to be the woman she wanted to be, independent of what she was doing each day.

She spent the time developing her sense of what it felt like to be in the field of Oneness, and in the field of fear. She noticed how many times a day she went back and forth, how many times she was triggered into an upset that she really would have preferred not to have.

In examining this, she began to see her preference for leaving the more drama-filled moments behind and finding her way into a more peaceful and compassionate relationship with life. She was seeing and beginning to choose the realm of life where she wanted to live. She was defining the source of her own reality.

As she chose to focus on the field of love, and bring her presence to her love intelligence, she created very important changes to her life. She felt free and expansive and able to make choices every day that supported her, specifically as it pertained to her sense of safety and love. And once having chosen her source, she was able to begin the process of defining specifics of her relationship to life for her personal culture. Of course she wasn't able to make this change permanently, but with her strong focus she was able to feel the tension coming on and practice bringing herself home. For the first time in her life, seeing this going back and forth between fields as a choice gave her the power to be who she wanted to be more and more.

So that is where we are starting today with you.

When after years of searching I got to this, it felt like a miracle to me. Maybe it is. You will tell me at the end of our time together if it does for you.

Who are you being? And who do you want to be today? Who are you proud of being? Are you living into that reality each day? Who does it feel good to be?

In this chapter I am offering you this solution, beyond the hope of life balance that will never come, a source that will guide you to your personal culture with life, a solution for the desperate feeling of an out of control life that is threatening to collapse around you. This solution provides you with a framework and structure to have in your life to make choices from. A personal culture that you will cultivate and immerse yourself in, one that will support you, one that will give you everything you need. You will be immersed in your own space in such a way as to no longer need opinions, rules, or outside pressure to find your truth and your way. You will have a sense of openness and therefore be available to true concerns and thoughts of people you trust in your life and still able to make your own decisions from your center about your life. This system is based in you and so is flexible as you grow and change over your life.

This solution is a sound one. It has been used many times, resulting in lives that are centered and whole, even within a busy life. It is practical and it is spiritual. As a minister, I will never give you a limited skill that will only work in a world you can see. This will also work in the realms that exist within you, whether you are familiar with them or not. It will touch you deeply and handle the everyday needs of your life. And it will take your commitment and work to do it.

At the end of the last chapter, you did an inventory. You looked to see what kind of personal culture is running in your life. And what the source of that is.

We begin where we are now – again, at your source of life. In this discussion I am attempting to assist in the understanding that no matter how many personal cultures there are, there are only two fields or sources that they can be based in, two sources for our lives. Personal cultures that are sourced from a field of duality, only create cultures that are forever choosing good/bad, right/wrong. These cultures are full of fear and instinctual behaviors and can be abusive, some are coddling, some are childish, some are dangerous, some are full of finger pointing and blame, some toward us and some toward others. These cultures usually embrace the stories of people as either victims or perpetrators. Neither person is helped in this consciousness.

As we discussed in the previous chapter, the field of duality is the field of fear. It is the basis of cultures of war, scarcity, force, and violence. These cultures are dualistic – there is right and there is wrong. They pit people against each other, and against the world. It leads only to more of the same, as it has only these things within its purview. When we choose fear, we will never be the highest expression of ourselves. We will always live bound by the most basic of mental constructs. We will struggle. We will be bound through our ancient nervous system to our fear. We cannot soar.

Still other cultures are sourced from a field of love or consciousness and can be seen in the lives of those who have decided to go beyond the norm and have a vision for more for their lives. Those cultures embrace nonviolence, restorative justice, compassion, caring, love and joy, abundance, creativity, and possibility.

If you choose fear, scarcity, and limitation as the basis for your personal culture, your source, that is what you will get in your life – and with it, usually a heavy dose of suffering, loneliness, and separation from others. I do not recommend this field. It is the default field of our sympathetic nervous system. Its bottom line is instinct and survival. In this field, we are always at war.

On the other hand is the unified field of oneness, love, and consciousness. It is the field where everything exists together in flow with each other and itself. Within this field, there is acceptance, compassion, love, and creativity. The endless possibilities of life exist and can be tapped to create the best life and the most joyful expression of ourselves ever. This is the field of our consciousness, our unlimited potential, our most expansive possibility.

You will have to choose one of these fields as your preference for the source of what you want to create, and who you want to be on your way.

Often the dreams for our lives are built in the field of love, but as we try to create them, we often slip into the field of fear with our worries, scarcity of resources, self doubt, and unmet needs and end up with a creation of scarcity, of shut down and dashed hopes and dreams. We don't see that we have changed our field, that our source has now shifted to fear, but it has.

When we try to create from the field of fear, we do not have access to what is necessary for us to create. As we begin to over-extend ourselves, we fall out of love. We lose our flexibility, our creativity, our light, and our breath. I am suggesting that the only way to live your dreams, to have the life you want without the pain and suffering, is to choose to step away from fear and into the field of loving and live in that field on your way.

In order to solve your overwhelm, your exhaustion, your fear of the loss of the dream of your life, choose love. When you choose this, you will be able to begin to reimagine the life you have always wanted and bring it to you with joy and creativity. And when you do, you will thereby be choosing the highest possibility for yourself and your life.

In some ways, this sounds easy. "Just let go, let things take care of themselves." Well, yes and no. It is simple and, you will need to completely reorient your life, your nervous system, letting go of your care for other's approval, your pettiness (hard to let go of), your unhealthy competitiveness, your manipulative games, just to mention a few. You will have to step out in trust, and listen and choose it before you can see it, because until you live it, it cannot show itself to you. If you are loving, you will feel and see love and if you have lived by controlling not trusting, that might be hard.

And, if you do choose love, it is not a permanent choice. The field of duality and fear will show up when it is triggered by fear. It is hard-wired into your brain, but, when you know what it is, you can choose again and again into the more expansive evolutionary reality of loving rather than being captured by fear and traveling down that endless downward spiral into darkness of fear and loss.

The unified field is our connection to all it is our loving source; this is a place where you will see miracles. This is the place where it will be possible for you to be the woman you want to be each day and live the life of your dreams.

Extraordinary States of Awareness

This is the place where we learn to trust our connection to life. This is where once we stop trying to control and demand and force life that we are released into where we can begin to see how things work naturally and fluidly together. From this consciousness we begin to take our foot off the gas and we let ourselves be guided by information that comes to us and information that flows through us in our relaxed and available state. We are opening up to the love intelligence within and surrounding us.

When life starts working this way it can be unsettling at first, but when we truly step in and allow ourselves to be supported and ask for our needs to be met from the Universe, miracles do happen. Life supports us and we find just what we need at just the right time.

This takes a while for people to understand and practice. It involves noticing all the serendipity or coincidences in our lives so we can begin to use all of the extraordinary information and guidance to make our lives easier. Once you start allowing yourself to use your internal guidance system, you will realize how much information you have been not seeing or hearing as you have focused only on that which is in form and seeable around you.

The gifts that come from insight, intuition, guidance, and knowing come to us all in different ways. Some of us see things or hear things that support us; mine comes in the form of a knowing. Suddenly I will know something, and then it will happen. And sometimes I have been wrong.

One of the ways this has worked for me in terms of staying out of overwhelm, is that when my days are full I still pace myself and breathe through tasks. I often will think of something make a quick call or run an errand and run into a person or find something that

I needed, saving me time or research on something that needed to get done. Another way this happens is that I will suddenly get an awareness of someone and when I turn my attention toward them something has happened or they need me or they are the right person to help me with a project. The more you live like this, the more your life flows with ease.

My life is full of moments of powerful knowing beyond the realm of what is palpable, as are the lives of my clients, family, and friends. As you get used to this, you begin to listen differently. This information is only available to you when you are trusting and in the field, when you are in a relaxed and open state.

When I was in my mid-thirties and had been studying with Mary and Ron Hulnick at the University of Santa Monica for a couple of years, I started to pay attention to this type of experience and guidance and begun tentatively to pay attention to it. This experience made me even more sensitive to these types of knowing.

I woke up one morning to the knowing that I was going to meet a man who was going to be very important in my life. I was going to meet him that day. It was a strange sensation in my body. I can still feel it and have now gotten more used to this way of knowing over the intervening years. That night I met three men and knew immediately he wasn't one of them, and at the very end of the night I saw a man as I left the room and my whole body shivered. I knew it was him. I decided to leave it until the next day to see what would happen. First thing the next morning, as I walked into the building, he was standing right in front of me. We talked for a moment and decided to meet upstairs after a few minutes. We were married a year and a half later, I step parented his children and we have a son together.

Now I am used to it. It is a great time saver as it delivers to me what I need in all sorts of forms every day. Even when I don't know I am looking for something.

I live from guidance with a loose plan for each day. Try it. You will never look back.

Let's get to work.

So while we have devoted a lot of space in this book to the discussion of source, it is not something we can go directly toward. It is something that whispers to us, it calls to us, it invites us through yearnings or talent or a leap of our hearts. This is the realm wherein all possibility exists. To be truly extraordinary, to not just live your life, but to live in a way that brings gifts to you and to many, we must cultivate this connection.

Our connection to source, to the ground on which we choose to stand, has nothing to do with religion, even though we can go through that portal to get there. It has nothing to do with what we have believed or what our experiences have been. Our connection to source is simply our deepest connection to life. It eventually becomes what we know.

On my journey, before I found this way to choose my source, I could feel a hollowness, a lack of some kind of meaning in my life, even though I thought I had everything. The truth is, I did have everything, everything I could think of.

But this world of source, this world is beyond thought. It exists in the imaginal realm; this is a realm of awakening, it is at the intersection of imagination and desire, it is not fantasy, it is an active part in the creation of your life. In order to have the best life, the most powerful, impactful, loving, or whatever you want, life, you will have to begin the journey within. That eventually will show you to you.

At this point in our journey you are going to spend some time in the field sourcing yourself, doing these practices over the next few days and perhaps some of them from now on. You need to have some experience in this field, and with how easily we either forget or get triggered out of it, in order for you to be able to choose your personal culture well. After you read the next two chapters, you will be acquainted with all of the areas of your personal culture and at the end of this section, we will gather and you will be invited to begin to outline your personal culture.

The Steps to Your Freedom

1. Sourcing Yourself from the Field of Oneness, Your Connection to the Universe

   Small steps continuously practiced with commitment open doors to the beauty within. We begin to try new things and listen to how we respond. These practices (we call them that because you will need to practice them) will take you into you, and to your wholeness beyond the specifics of you.

   - *Meditation* of any kind begins to slow you and invite you to connect within. The simplest starting meditations of sitting for one minute quietly and observing your thoughts can begin a lifelong love affair with yourSelf. Meditation also includes many kinds of breathing and slow gentle movement practices, letting your eyes rest gently on the light of a candle, and many other simple practices to focus your mind, and let go as well. There are many resources for developing deeper experience, but really what it takes, is just doing it. It is meant to be a simple practice. That does not make it easy.

   - *Contemplation* is a practice of reading inspirational material, religious or otherwise, poetry or anything that is uplifting, and then allowing yourself the space and time to really deeply ponder the ideas and wonder with curiosity if they feel like truth to you.

   - *Movement* that is in alignment with your body, either self-chosen movements or following a class or a teacher. Walking, dancing, allowing yourself to feel into what delights you. What brings more life to you? Yoga, ecstatic dance, Tai Chi, and many more practices are available for you to explore. What moves you? As it moves you, it will move your spirit.

- *Experiencing the natural world* is an important practice to ground ourselves in nature and feel the connection that we have to the earth. It can be as simple as couple of minutes with shoes off on the grass in front of your office, or as complex and extravagant as a week away in Bimini (of course I recommend the week away anywhere!)

- *Writing* in your journal could include practices of unedited expression, or gratitude, musings, or expansive thoughts about what you want, dreams, hopes, fears… all of it begins to open the door to you. Some of us are writers and some not. I wrote for years and woke up one day and could no longer make myself write in a journal. Instead, I create idea maps on my phone after meditating.

- *Engaging your creativity* is one of the best ways to find your center, your place at home with yourself. For some it is sewing, for some cooking, for some design, for some paint or photos and, well, you get the idea – find what you love.

- And don't be surprised if something new shows up. I became a poet in this practice after a year of journaling, which gave me an outlet for my grief and being able to place it in a bigger context after my sister died.

- Here, within, I became whole again.

- Another thing that may show up is that you will be presented with parts of you that want to heal as you sit, move, create, or journal.

- *Healing and forgiveness* may come to you as well as an opportunity to let go of something that hurt you but is not you, and return you to wholeness again.

Most importantly, we invite ourselves into a conversation of love and acceptance with anything that hurts within us. We do our best to see and let go of our wounds and hurts, and then forgive ourselves and others as we can.

Your personal culture with life:

Some of your best ideas will come to you in the quiet of this place as you develop comfort and you begin to feel yourself there. In this quiet place of patience and kindness to yourself, you will find your deepest self. And you will find the reward is greater than you will have imagined. As you begin to define this place where you reside in joy and self-expression, you will begin to define you. You will learn to turn within and seek your deepest answers from your source and your sense of yourself.

This will lay the groundwork for your opening to the expansion that is available to you through your relationship with yourself and what you perceive as your place in the Universe. This connecting does not need to take much time; each one of these activities are possible from one minute to hours. That is up to you. In the beginning consistency especially matters, not necessarily the length of time engaged in the activity.

From your source, you will be feeling into a sense of who you are in relationship to the whole of life and what you want in your life. This is where your personal culture with Life is born. As you are connecting to your source, you will be finding your way into a sense of how you want to participate with life. As you do that, you don't need to define every bit of your personal culture, just what is necessary to begin to build your foundation of your life from being centered here in love. In this realm sourced from love, part of the magic is being present to what wants to happen or simply following where you are led as you surrender the need to know all the time.

How will you know you are there or have been there?

Signposts of being sourced in the unified field, of love:

- You will experience a sense of spaciousness or out-of-timeness with the regular pace of your life.
- You will enjoy a sense of calm and connection that gives you a sense of being at home in yourself.
- You will have moments of intuition and insight that are beyond what you are capable of "thinking" of on your own.
- You will begin to have a sense of peace and joy in your day.
- You will be less harried and worried. More full of grace in many ways.
- You will sense peace within you. Your breath will relax and you will feel coherence with the Universe.

2. Choosing Your Source: It's up to You

   The choice is now yours. How will you proceed? What will you choose and how will it define your life?

   If you choose fear, survival, or scarcity, you will still have a good life. You will still have things you want and people who love you. And, you may not even be aware of how it might be limiting you, so if you find a time when things feel stagnant and small, come back to this chapter and consider it all again. I actually suggest that you come back to that choice often. You may see specific areas in your life where you will choose this field and other areas where you choose love.

   It is all perfectly fine and you can do the rest of this book that way. And, you may find that it is easier and more fun and faster to get what you want if you let this go and step in fully to the field of love and your love intelligence.

   In either case, I support your choice and the dignity of your process. You are autonomous and that is what our ultimate freedom is all about.

If you choose love, this is an expansion choice. The treasures will be yours to mine and use in your life. You will be able to choose to be the person you want to be as you do these practices with consistency and commitment. You will be evolving you through the dynamic connection between you and source. You will be growing you. And feeling the power inherent in that choice.

This is the time when it is up to you to choose. Will you avail yourself of these practices? Will you immerse yourself in this field and find your way home to love? Will you choose to see life as an experience of oneness?

If you choose the field of love, you will spend the rest of your life learning and growing in all the ways that you can find to expand into the release necessary to choose this field. This is not a choice that is for the faint of heart. It requires seeing beyond what others see, it requires trust to an unheard of degree. And, it will pay you well. Simple. Not easy.

Intrinsic in this choice is the automatic failure introduced every time we get scared. The work is to remember this choice even when we get off center so we may come back more quickly and reliably to our center and our peace.

As you do the practices above, there will be things inside you that will be forced to the surface – wounds, pain, addictions, fears, and hurts. But this is the work of the evolution of our humanity, our compassion, and our brains. This is the work of healing through the application of loving to everything. That is integrity. That is love.

"Your task is not to seek for love, but merely to seek and find all the barriers within yourself that you have built against it."
                                    – Jalāl ad-Din Huhammad Balkhi ~ Rūmi

CHAPTER 6

You with *You*

The second component of the process of defining your personal culture is your relationship with you. How do you see yourself in your life? What do you think of yourself – what are the needs and desires that you have? This is a deeply sacred process of inviting you into an awareness of how you hold yourself in relationship to you in your life. These are big questions and when answered can give us all sorts of leverage to create with. You will be invited into a new way to find yourself, to support yourself in having what it takes to live a happy, joy-filled life that is full of responsibilities, people, and challenges without having to give your life away to have all that. And by doing your part you will find yourself having people who love and care for you assist you in having it all.

You see, what I am going to provide you with here is an opportunity to transform who you are being in any situation (like when you are upset and yelling or being silent and unrelenting or worse) by transforming where you are coming from, the source of who you are. And in showing you that when you are doing that, you are being here for you.

You show up for you. Yes, there will be circumstances for which we will need others but first, are you willing to put yourself first? Are you willing to show up for you?

I am suggesting that the most important thing that you can learn from this is that you must put yourself and your needs first. Before anything or anyone else.

We must take the strongest stand for this as you are the only one accountable for yourself. And you, having been made in the image and likeness of the divine, must be divine. You are holy, and as such must treat yourself and your needs so.

You must be willing to take a stand for yourself, who you are, and put everything on the line for yourself and for your needs to be met. This will prove to be a generous and kind act if you want to be in partnership with others. This is the only way your relational partnerships will survive. You must be here. You must be present, and you must be cared for so you can be available. To offer the best of who you are, you must be the best of who you are. You must choose to treat yourself as the one that you are solely responsible for. You take exquisite care of you, and you are then, and only then, able to give without conditions to those around you.

In our lives, we sometimes choose to try to fix things on the surface only and not get to the root of what is happening. In this chapter, we are going to look into you. We are going to look into who you are capable of being when you are full, supported, and giving from your overflow, and who you are being when you are tired, spent, overworked, overwhelmed, judging yourself, or pushing yourself, to name a few of the strategies we use to get ourselves to do things … and then what happens when we don't take care of ourselves.

For instance, if you are living in a world where you are taking care of your needs, getting to self-care classes, having fun, feeling appreciated at work, sexy at home, and fun, you might be full. If so, you will have within you kindness and peace and have plenty of time and space and when someone asks you to help them with something, you (like me) will probably be able to assist, even be happy to assist. If your values line up with wanting to have partnerships that work, and you care for the asker, you will probably assist them.

But, if you feel full and crowded with too many unmet needs of your own, with too many responsibilities, with resentments, anger, and overwhelming responsibilities – we all know what will happen if someone asks for some assistance, especially if it is one of the people you love and care for the most. The sentence starts with something like "Are you kidding me?" and goes off from there....

So, what if, what if you could choose to give the best care to yourself and support yourself in where you are coming from all the time? What if that choosing will give you to you everyday? What if you do not have to strategize and demand and manipulate to get support and care for yourself? What if you create it all so that you have ways of caring for yourself that make it so you can be available and have overflow to give from?

This is part of living the dream. And you can do this.

As we go back over the material from the last couple of chapters and focus again on how we get you into the field of love and consciousness, if we are to be partners on this journey I am really going to need your help.

Actually, it is going to be up to you to do your part.

Here is your first question.

What do you need to be you? Your best you?

First: a need is something that you get a big benefit from if met or a big loss if not. Something that will make you happy counts! We are working here to return you to yourSelf.

What if with all the good intentions in the world you can't be you without getting your needs met?

What would you commit to? What needs do you really need, in which areas of your life?

As soon as you are not getting what you need, you are sacrificing. As soon as you are sacrificing, you are no longer capable of partnership and accessing the field of love. You are immediately enrolled in the dualistic field of fear/scarcity/instinct and conflict.

Can you see it? I could. When I first learned this I was stunned. It made so much sense. As soon as I sacrifice, I am out of partnership and in a mode in which I am operating at a deficit. When I am doing that. I am lost. We are lost and in big trouble for being able to navigate the regular day, much less stormy waters in some upset. Probably no one will ever get it right for you. Why?

Because *you* are not there. You have left the field as soon as your need was not met. You are no longer in the game anymore. You have left. All that you have left behind is your upset, needy, angry instinctual self. You, yourself, have been lost. Your relationship with yourself and with others will sink from this.

Who you are, the Self that you are working hard at being, cannot survive without you protecting her and her needs. You cannot give up on her. She needs you, the world needs her. She must have those needs met.

Look in these areas:
- *Physical*: your home, your office – do they reflect you or distract you? How is your health? Your exercise? Your food? Your sleep? Today? Overall?
- *Mental*: how is your mind? Are you balanced or distracted?
- *Emotional*: are you overwhelmed or on the edge all the time? Are you feeling cared for?
- *Spiritual*: are you connected to your essence in source or are you in the field of fear and separation, slugging it out, with effort and a desire to control?

Take some time and really look at what you need. Every moment. Every day. Every week. Every month.

Remember, without you taking care of yourself first, you can't source your life, and you can't be yourself. It is your job and service to the world to make sure you are doing this first.

We will look into this more in the later chapter about your presence, but it is good to take a look now.

Once you have looked this over, look to see what needs you actually need someone else's help to satisfy. The ones you can't meet all by yourself.

What do you need that you need partnership with someone in your life fulfill. Now, I am sure you can imagine that when I started working on this list for myself, it got to be very long. So we are going to give you a caveat. Here it is. Your partners, in this case, your husband, your kids, your helpers and assistants, all have lives and jobs of their own. So while we understand that you have lots to do, you must watch the tendency to give too much away and then have a team of very exhausted, resentful people around you. So, stick to less than five needs that you need support fulfilling for now. Also, we are not asking these people to provide all of it, just what you need – the part that you can't create for yourself without their partnership.

That might look like, you need a good night's sleep and you have kids. So you might need a couple nights in a row of going to bed at 8 p.m. and not being interrupted all night. Let's say you ask your husband for this. You would check in with him to see if he feels he can provide that for you.

Here is a tricky part.

In *relational partnerships* there are a couple of guidelines:

1. If they are able, your loving partner will give you what you ask for because they love and care for you and they want you to be happy – as long as it *does not* require any (nada, nothing, not) *sacrifice* on their part. In other words,

if your husband is going to go without sleep, this is not okay. You might have to get an overnight nanny, doula, or some such. Clear?

2. If your partner says "No," you accept that no. That does not mean you can't change something to see if your partner is willing, but you do not wheezily whine, get angry, blame, or shoot the one who says no. Got it? Good. Tactics used by others to get a yes after a no has been issued (possibly by the author, but I'm not admitting anything) include dressing scantily, plying one's partner with alcohol, promising favors or any such nonsense that "no one ever has ever done." Check yourself on this and don't come back with a "No! Me? Never!" If you get that answer, try again. This time, ask, "When did I use a tactic like this to turn my partner's solid no into the yes I wanted?" Slow down a second and let your brain show you. It will. Now you got it? We all do it. We are not proud of it. It is part of our being human when we are sourced in fear.

3. Giving up your need because someone can't provide what you asked them for is *not okay*. Yes, you heard that right. Just because your partner cannot provide for your need does not mean that you give that up. You just told us it was so important to you that you need partnership to get it. Do not, I repeat, do not give it up. What could happen? Anger, resentment, destruction of your relational partnership. Do you need more reasons? If you really need it, you really need it.

One of the bottom line tenets of this type of partnership is that *unmet needs create havoc and so they are not okay*.

I did not say you can only have five needs. I said, you can only have five needs that you are getting partnership to create. This is obviously different in the case of an employee who is your direct report.

You can have as many needs as you have. You are responsible for those, it's just that you are only going to ask for partnership on the ones you cannot meet by yourself.

You are ultimately responsible for getting all your needs met. If someone cannot give it to you, you will have the chance to find someone else, or change the form of your partnership in order to get your need met.

In a short aside, there are many ways to handle this. For example, you are not satisfied in your sex life. You have sex once a year and it is always mediocre. It feels like your partner feels like it is a chore and you are really unhappy about it. (We are going to start with the assumption that a good sex life is a real need, if it is for you.)

A possible scenario could be: your husband is unwilling to provide sex but you love him and your family *and* you need to have a sexual partnership. You could a) keep your marriage intact and have a lover on the side or b) you could choose another type of partnership with your husband that keeps the family intact but dissolves the marriage so you are free to find someone else as your primary partner. You could date multiple people – anything that is okay with both partners will keep the partnership alive and keep creating from love, honor, and respect. And, even if you don't reach an agreement, an agreement to keep partnership alive can produce miraculous results.

Okay, so you have five things. Five things? Yes. So think long and hard about this. How will you prioritize? How will you choose?

Many new parents sacrifice sleep. And we see so many completely stressed families because of it. Many divorces have come about from non-sleeping parents in families that don't solve their need for sleep.

What are the things you go without? If you are stressed overworked, overwhelmed, and overtired, what needs have you not taken care of?

This is a powerful important and undervalued issue in partnership with yourself and with others. It must be addressed.

What do you need in order to be You?

Some things that people have big needs around:

- Helpers
- Sex
- Sleep
- Food
- Health
- Partner's health
- Finances
- Spending
- Kids (food, health, emotional health, school....)
- Vacations
- Work

... you get the idea

Start working on the list of everything you need. Have fun, take your time, enjoy the process, and go for it. All of it.

Specify how many times a week and how long.

Go: *(e.g., eight hours of sleep a day, two hours of swimming a week, three yoga classes a week, five walks a week; one at the beach. Two hours each weekend day to myself. One hour a night for brainless TV after the kids are in bed. Two nights a week in which I don't put the kids to bed, one romantic date night out of the house a week ....)*

Your short list for your partners: The five things you need that you cannot do without a partnership contribution in your life.

Include: "Who is your partner in this?" and "What is your need?" are your job. "How it will get done?" is your partner's choice, better to stay out of that.

GO:

1._____

2.————————————————————

3.————————————————————

4.————————————————————

5.————————————————————

And, now think of the things that are on your list that you have been hanging on to, things that maybe you want, maybe you have been being hard on someone else for not providing for you. You may have just realized that they are only sort of important, you haven't even committed to them for yourself, or they are something you actually can do for yourself but you don't want to, and maybe you've not even asked for them because, well, "everyone knows" that should be provided for you – five things to let go of that are not that important (make a list, ladies, and work up from the bottom). Some ideas – he should call you every day from work, pick up your cleaning when he's out, clean your car once a week, open the door for you, take the kids right when he gets home, not need you for....

1.————————————————————

2.————————————————————

3.————————————————————

4.————————————————————

5.————————————————————

And of course, reciprocate this with all your partners.
Bless you, your partnerships will thank you.

CHAPTER 7

Love Others as Much as You Love Yourself

O thers. Singleness. Here, I am introducing the concept that we are mirrors of each other through projection, our inevitable realization that we are all made of the same material and as such all one. If you see something in another, it already resides in you. We are all cut from the same cloth and we are all in this life, world, environment, and Universe together. We will be able to see the value that it is to us as we learn to treat others in a way that reflects our highest values and desires and see how that will impact our partnerships.

Some of us can't create partnership with anyone. Some of us can create partnership with some but not most. Some of us can make alliances with family, friends, colleagues, and lovers. That can feel like partnership, but at some point we eventually sort out that alliances are inherently adversarial; the moment there is a threat to the alliance each will turn against the other and/or go their separate ways. These won't establish long-lasting friendships, partnerships, or ties of any kind. When there is pressure, they will break.

Until we claim each other fully as ourselves we will always be involved to some degree in the game of us versus them, good versus bad – any duality that serves to keep us separate will never serve our highest purpose.

Some of us make peace in our hearts, with ourselves, and then in our families, and on the most rare of occasions some of us will share that with the world. When we truly do that, eventually we realize that true partnership is partnership within the wholeness of who we are. Not everyone will give us the partnership in the day-to-day that we want and that will give us the chance to choose a different sort of partnership with them, but we do not need to shatter partnership in and of itself.

As we look to our spiritual roots, we are offered the possibility of not separating from even the ones who don't want to participate with us, by offering them our willingness to hold them in a place of acceptance for the dignity of their process, and the innocence of their deepest self. This kind of partnership is not something that you will participate within your daily life except perhaps in your spiritual practice, but it is the only way for us to achieve wholeness. If wholeness is so, none must be condemned outside our wholeness.

It's a tricky conversation but I trust you are savvy well enough to know what we are speaking of here or at least to trust that we will find our way to deeper understanding. I cannot help or heal or bring myself in love in my life if I am judging and closing my heart to even one other. Why? Because the field we need to access is a unified field. You cannot negotiate with that. It is created that way and can only function that way. There is no changing that.

At the deepest level of source, if we look for innocence, we will find it, first in ourselves and from there, in others. There is a sense of the possibility of partnership with all people, all beings, all life, and the cosmos. This is not easy to do but it is the foundation of all partnerships, so must be explored. First, we will guide you through the personal level, and then to the fuller experience of your wholeness through all types of partnership.

As we enter the third realm of relational partnership sourced from the field, we consider the role of others in the way we carry ourselves in life.

In the previous chapter, while we involved our partners, we were still focused on ourselves.

The theory that we are one with each other gives us a unique way of seeing ourselves. This is something that a lot of people struggle with. It is a psychological key to who we are that we hide from ourselves. Because we can't see our blind spots, we are vulnerable to being sidelined by them. Our partners offer us a simple, easy way to see ourselves. All we need to do is find ourselves upset with them for any reason, and we can begin to delve inside.

Projection is an idea based in the principle that whatever we don't want to see in ourselves, we give to another and can therefore see it more clearly. The problem arises because we most often think it really is the other person who is causing our upset, and let's be honest, sometimes what they are doing doesn't work, but the "causing upset" part is the part for us to look at.

We are now stepping into an awareness of who we are with our partners, who we want to be with them, and what is possible as we embrace the power of having a shared mission, a combined vision of what we want to create in our lives. What is possible when we become a team.

As we look at our partners through this lens of this paradigm, we see the necessity of understanding that not only does it seem like we are in this life together, and not only does it in fact happen that we are in this life together, but that there is something much more powerful about how we are connected than that.

When we really understand that our partners are our commitments, not our allies, our friends, or our sparring partners, we begin
to understand the importance of the concept of singleness, of oneness.

When we consider that the truth that is held in this paradigm is
not that we are like each other, or even that we are connected, it is
much deeper. It is that we are one. And how that plays out in relational partnerships is miraculous.

As soon as you remember that your partner is you, and while he
is special and unique differently than you, he is nonetheless special
and unique, and, he gives you a chance to be the best person you can
be. He gives you the opportunity to be your best self, every day. The
beauty of our partners is that they are always serving our evolution
by helping us to see ourselves, not as we want to see ourselves, but
as we really are.

We look into the face of our partners and what we see that looks
like their flaws are really just gifts giving us a chance to see our own
flaws, giving us a chance to look for the love and the goodness that
is there within us instead of the demands of perfection.

Partnerships thrive when both partners see their reflection in
each other and in so doing, see themselves, take ownership, and
give themselves to the love present for healing, instead of to the
judgments and blame that will pull them further apart.

The beautiful system that exists in this universe is that we are
going to find a way to attract the very person who we need to support us to learn and grow the most. Sometimes our soul partners are
the hardest ones to live with, especially when we don't want to learn
and grow.

As we look at own our own reflection, heal our pain, own our
own innocence, and act to bring more love to the surface, the world
becomes a better place.

Treating others the way we want to be treated has been said in
a million different ways in languages the world over; we call it the

Golden Rule. The limitation of the way it is usually expressed is often that the one who is giving is led to believe that it is good and holy and perhaps even a better gift if the giver sacrifices to the one they are giving to.

As we know from our work in the last chapter, that is not a healthy, sustainable system. The only way the system works is if we are indeed one, and the putting ourselves first that we talked about in the previous chapter then pertains to each other, and then to the rest of the world.

As we take on a world where partnership works, we take on a world where it is possible to hold a grand vision for peace on this planet through peace in ourselves, our partnerships, and our families.

As we stop looking at each other across the great divide of what seems like a chasm of difference between people and instead, look for that which is the same, the humanity that we share, that which when we look clearly give us the deepest level of respect for ourselves and each other. We will be free.

As we perceive others, one of the most important tasks is to see with kindness and accuracy. We must put down the swords embedded in our stories, the daggers in our assumptions of guilt, and the knives we wield in our blame; all these are the weapons of our unforgiveness.

If we look clearly with kindness, we will see each person's innocence, each person's need. We will see that action taken is always held within the reasoning of what we think at the time we act. When we think with judgment, with rancor toward others, with revenge for wrongdoing, we will be that. And we will never heal ourselves, our world, or each other.

We must think with innocence. It delivers us from the need to judge and slay others with our twisted untruths.

We are indeed from one source, and as such we are the same, and as we are the same, we follow the Golden Rule to the source and we see, we are one. As I treat myself as the child of the Universe, as holy as the Universe itself, I bow to you as I see you are me in this knowing.

When we take on this deeper message of love, respect, honor and care, kindness, patience, and compassion, we give it equally to ourselves and to each other.

When we find ourselves in the most mundane of circumstance, circling the drain, doubting our partner's love and sincerity, we must turn and look again within ourselves.

That is where our life lies. We step fully into the power of owning our shadow, our stories, our darkness, and we are free in an instant to let them go.

So for now, we look to our partners with grace and we say, I am the light of the world and I see that in you as well. I bow to me as I bow to you. We are one.

As we take on this practice of seeing ourselves in our partners, our children, our lovers, and our enemies, as we let go, we can release the walls of separation and step out into a world of love and freedom.

A world where everything works.

For our partnerships when there is this much love and respect, when anything we give to ourselves is also seen as integral to others, we will be free.

How Are We Going to Get There?

I am going to tell you a story and go through this process with you, then you can do it yourself applying it to something in your life. I am going to use an example of a couple I worked with but this is the same process you do with anyone in your life that you are partnering with.

In this chapter, we are going to ask you to be the best partner you can be by trying this on. It is hard, I'm not gonna lie, but you can do it.

First, I am going to give you an example and then a template for you to try it.

Think of a Time When Something Happened

Michael would get up on Saturday morning, read the paper, have breakfast with the kids, and then head out to the gym. He would sometimes hang out a little or do something on the way home so he would come home later than Martha wanted him to.

Make up Your Story

Martha's story was that Michael was not pulling his weight with the family. He was spending too much time on himself and wasn't helping her get her needs met. She had had the kids all week while he was traveling, and she needed some time to herself and some space to get away. He was selfish and he didn't care about her well-being. He didn't care about her or the kids. It was all about him.

Tell the Story

When Martha told me this story it was very clear that she was very upset with Michael. They both had big jobs and it always seemed like she was left "holding the bag" of care on Saturday for the animals and the kids and sorting out the day while he went out to take care of himself. She was really angry and even more so because she felt like it really showed a lack of caring for her. That was her biggest complaint.

Feel the Story

As she began to tell me the story, she started to cry. She told me how much she felt like she gives to him and the family. She was just barely keeping it together and then, just when she would think she was going to get relief, instead of supporting her or helping her, Michael would just leave her and go and take care of himself. At this point, she was really more angry than sad. She expressed both and I had lot of empathy for her – she was really hurting. And in expressing her feelings, she was beginning to feel more herself again.

Taking Some Space: Breathe, Move, Tell the Truth to Yourself

Since I do a lot of client work on the telephone, we agreed to take a break here and she would go do something for herself to connect with herself. She promised not to communicate with Michael until she did her work and felt better. After she was back in herself (connected with her source, away from fear) then she would talk to Michael about what had happened and all that was up for her.

Find out the Truth from Your Partner

When she talked to Michael later in the day she was calm and centered. When they did talk, she asked him to tell her about Saturdays and what he liked and wanted. A funny thing happened, because she gave him some space and he wasn't at all defensive – he told her how he likes to get his workout done so he can be there to run the kids around later and give her a break for as much of the day as possible, plus she was better at the organizing the kids and parent thing so he figured he was just in the way…. She was stunned. The truth he was operating under was completely different than she was assuming it was! They talked a little longer and she was able to ask him to support her a little differently sometimes. He was agreeable, no fight, no bad.

Now it is time to turn our attention back to Martha.

What about Your Stories Is About You?

As she looked at the story she had made up, and how different it was from Michael's experience or what he was doing, she realized that something in all this was going on in her. And so we looked.

She was hurting. That was true. The thing that bothered her the most was that she felt like he didn't care about her and that he was showing up with such a lack of care for her. She looked at her judgment of Michael as uncaring and dismissing her needs and then looked to see how those things were true for her. She saw that she really was the one who was not planning time for herself or caring for herself. She was leaving it for other people to provide for her, and, because she was so depleted, she could not even see that he was leaving most of the day for her to take care of what she needed. She realized she needed to be taking better care of herself.

Relook for Innocence

In this situation, she was able to immediately see the innocence in Michael's actions, and beyond that, in the care that he thought he was providing. It was so great that they did not have to waste time in arguing or upsetting the kids. She was so grateful.

Do You Need Something?

She did decide that while she loved Michael's thoughtfulness, what she really wanted was Saturday mornings to herself.

Ask

When she went home, she asked her husband for the Saturday mornings that she wanted. She did it from a place of appreciation for what he had already done, and just asked if they could try something differently that would support her better. And she asked him if there was anything he needed to support that for her.

Commitment to Take Care of You with Feedback, and Without Sacrifice

To this, Michael responded that he would like to try Martha's suggestion on a Saturday and see how it went. He didn't know how it would be for him and would like some room to try again if he needed something different. He asked her if she would be willing to remind him on Friday night so he wouldn't forget and disappoint her.

Martha was happy to start there.

Home

They took a few moments to look into each other's eyes. Martha was able to share authentically with Michael what she had felt and what she had learned about herself and her own self-care. In this moment, they had established a very sweet connection between them and acknowledged the love and care they had for themselves and each other. They felt at home together in an intimate caring place. Both at home in the field of love.

The Template for You

Think of a Time When Something Happened

What was the actual thing that happened, not all the other stories you built up around it? Only the facts. What can you see?

Think of a Story

… of a time when something happened and, without checking it out, you decided you for sure knew what was going on? (Your husband was being lazy, the kids don't even care about you, even the dog loves everyone else more …).

Tell the Story

… details, feelings, thoughts, everything.

Taking Some Space

Breathe and go for a walk, get a coffee... do something to support yourself.

Feel the Story

How did you feel after you told your story?

What did you make up about the other people or the situation?

Breathe, Move, Tell the Truth

Are you willing to slow down and get this process going when you both have created time and space to breathe, connect, and work together to resolve this?

Find Out the Truth

What really was going on? (You may have to leave this blank until later when you find out there might be some inaccuracies in your story.)

What about Your Stories Is About You?

Can you see your judgments? (Lazy, stupid, entitled, etc.)

How are those things true about you? (Even if you don't like the idea or see it, consider it. You can come back later if you can't do it now.)

Relook

Can you begin to see the innocence in the other person's choice of action?

Do You Need Something?

Do you need something specific to be different? Do you know the other person doesn't have to give it to you?

Have you told them that?

Ask

Have you told the other person what it will give you to receive the gift of their partnership around this?

With honor and respect for the life and personality and needs of others in the situation, what is already going on in their life? What do they need? Please ask.

Do you see that you are asking for partnership in your need? Do you see that they may not have the same need?

Commitment to Take Care of You with Feedback, and without Sacrifice

Do you see that the other person will do this for you if they can? And not if they have to sacrifice?

(How do you usually "get" what you need? When someone first says no?)

Even though that frustrates you, do you understand that the other person's truth is important in creating a solution that works from partnership and not from demand, manipulation, threats, or bribes?

Can you see that their authentic response might save you from falling into a hole with your solution?

Home

Create a closing ritual and check-in if you need to repair or heal anything together.

Great work. I love you. You are coming back to *you*.

You are awesome. Your life and *you* are growing together. Not easy. Not for sissies, but are you one? I didn't think so. You've got this.

You are here to change the world. Start with you, your close partnerships, and then the world. Thank you for your commitment.

We can't do it without you.

CHAPTER 8

Personal Culture – Creating the Field of You

The premise that we are working from is that when you are sourced in truth and love, your life moves with guidance and surrender into a form that is perfectly suited for you. That what has been hard and painful and disturbing and uncomfortable can be healed and released. And as your field gets clearer and clearer, your life will flow with grace, harmonize with resonance, and fill your world with light.

The reason that is important is that in order to live a full and powerful life, you must surrender your attempt to control it. The more you try to control your life, the more you micro manage people in your life, the more you won't let go and let things flow, the more stagnant you will be and the less you will actually be able to get done.

Overwhelm is birthed in the wheelhouse of control, fear, scarcity, forcing, pushing, demanding, and manipulating for what you think is best and will keep you safe. The more you do this, the more alone you actually are. The more alone you are, the less effective you are. We live in a dynamic system that is highly creative, loving and here for you.

When you embrace that, act on that, live with that as your reality, you will be free. Your life will flow, things will come to you. You will have the assistance of the entire Universe and all the people you need to get things done.

As long as you remain yourSelf.

Now that we have the three components of personal culture discussed, it is time to create a personal culture that will stand with you for now and is flexible enough that it can be changed and updated in time.

This is an important place to really spend some time with yourself. A strategy that might be helpful would be to go back over the chapters and reconnect with yourself and your material.

Most importantly, start with yourself, and start connected to your source and to yourself.

This is the place to center in and very deeply consider what you want to be when you are your *best* self. Really consider it.

It is time to create the field of you, your personal culture.

Your best self: the life of you. The ideal experience of you with source, yourself, and others in your life.

Your Experience of Source

Who can you be when you are sourced in love? Are you willing to practice letting go of fear? (You won't always be able to do it.)

Who are you when you are sourced in fear?

Choose your Source: Love or Fear.

Creating Your Personal Culture

1. Qualities of being that you are committed to in partnership with *life*: *Who* you are committed to being, no matter what. (Until you mess up and then commit again.)

What are you committed to creating in relation to life itself and the world you live in? What are your values, what do you want to contribute? Love, compassion, kindness, creativity.

2. Qualities of being that you are committed to in partnership with *you*: Who you are committed to being in relation to yourself?

    What are you committed to creating in your personal world for you? What are your values? Calm environment, self-attention in meditation, honor, kindness, compassion.

3. Qualities of being that you are committed to in partnership with *others*: Who you are committed to being in relation to others in your world? What are your values, what do you want to contribute? Kindness, patience, grace, honor, inclusiveness, acceptance

    What are you committed to creating in your family/work and social world? What are your values, what do you want to contribute? Flow and grace, love and peace, fun

    What are you committed to creating in your community? What are your values, what do you want to contribute? Local politics, community building, sharing resources, raising loving children.

    What else are you committed to creating in the larger world. What are your values, what do you want to contribute? World peace, expansion, empowerment ….

LQ: Love Intelligence:
Part 3 –

How to Get What
You Need from Everyone

CHAPTER 9
Work, Children, Love, and Sex

*"Mastery in the art of living makes little distinction
between work and play, labor and leisure, mind and body,
information and recreation, love and religion. Mastery
means hardly knowing which is which. Simply pursue a
vision of excellence at whatever you do, leaving others to
decide whether you are working or playing. In the field of
mastery, you know you're always doing both."*
– (adapted from) James A. Michener

I would venture to say, that mastery in the art of living has within
it, in the hidden realms, the attempt at mastery in the art of relational partnerships. As you may have noticed, I won't even venture to say that mastery in relational partnerships is possible. But the
pursuit of mastery is the critical thing.

I have pursued this avenue of living with caring for and loving
the people in my life, but, earlier in my life, I had missed the crucial
distinction that all people are people in my life. I compartmentalized

some, leaving them out of the center of my care, often leading them to feel dishonored, disrespected, and not valued. This learning led me to see the power of offering partnership to all people in our lives, offering a working together that works within the flexible parameters of partnership with my life and mySelf and together with others in every part of my life.

It is not as we might have thought in the past, that our relationships that matter are only the ones we have with our primary loved ones, at home and separate from what we do all day as we work. Or that we create relationships in different compartments or areas of our lives and there is no contact of interrelating them. Now we see the potent possibility that there is no place where love cannot be found and enhance our experience if we are looking for it. And we must look. In order to be all that we want, to live a full life and feel the fulfillment of aliveness, we must look for love within, around and between us and others.

In the suggestion made by Michener in the quote about work and play at the beginning of this chapter, I would guess that the critical ingredient that makes work and play in this instance the same as each other is the relational partnerships underneath them. All doing (work or play) is the same if the source of them both, what is underneath them, is love.

The distinction we are making between relationships and relational partnerships is an important one. We are suggesting that relationships just happen. They are brought on and let go of by factors that mainly have to do with attraction and repulsion from our instinct to connect to live. That is a survival game and usually ends in a control battle for who will be the predator, and who the prey. Going back to our conversations about being sourced from fear, survival, or scarcity, you probably remember this.

Relationships do not have within them any inherent skill set nor ability to understand ourselves and each other and care for each other well. On the contrary, we are most often leading from survival, the need to connect to stay alive, the need to procreate, the need to have status, which leaves us mostly in a dog-eat-dog world, without what is necessary to keep us in good shape to be the best that we can be in those relationships. This is the problem I ran into in my marriage in Chapter 2.

We are establishing a personal culture on the other hand, and teaching a way of being that creates powerful loving in your life, with yourSelf, and with one another. Your Love intelligence or LQ will be high is a result of learning and some mastery of choosing loving consciousness as your source, implementing and abiding in the three key components of your personal culture, and participating with these four basic LOVE ingredients of partnership.

Without commitment to your source, living your personal culture and practicing the ingredients of partnerships, the process of life and the pull of fear will land you squarely back floundering, sacrificing, demanding, and manipulating for any love you can get. Those alliances are based in fear: giving to get and taking to have, manipulating to appease, contorting to please, and overpowering to handle our needs. Sound familiar? Yes, we do it every day.

Our survival system is hardwired so we will keep going back into those ancient sources of fear where our unhealthy behaviors come from. And then we are lost. We end up alone, doing life alone, feeling alone. From here we have created a false safety one that will end up taking us away from the mastery that we want, and into the pain of loneliness and separation.

So, I again suggest, that the attempt at mastery in relational partnership is worth the effort, sourcing us in the field of love, beyond survival and instinct to a place where relational partnerships exist, is worth all the preparation. Every moment spent in shared experience of loving is taking you further into your life toward what you want than any other path you will travel and guiding you toward fulfillment on the way.

"When all our labor is a labor of love, then all our life is Love. That is Mastery."

We experience our relationships moment by moment, or even experience by experience. The more we love the more we feel it, the more we feel it, the more we become it. It is a journey of discovery and it makes life an adventure of love each day.

When all your life is lived in love and with partnership, you will have turned the key in the lock and opened the door to you and your full experience of life and stepped fully into your freedom, happiness, and expanded possibility.

The Hidden Component: Accountability

It is now possible for you to step into partnership with everyone.

And I mean that. Everyone. Now that you are a student of relational partnerships, everyone is your new potential partner. You and the Universe, you and yourself, and you and others, the planet, and the community of life. You choose from you.

This process of relational partnership for human beings is not meant to be carried out in perfection. Partnership it is meant to be creative, held and looked at, considered, and wondered about. And even after that, re-shaped to fit you and used with the basic building blocks of your personal culture as support.

This journey you have embarked on is sacred. It is about giving commitments to life and doing your best to care for yourself first, along with others on the way.

Accountability and the elements of LQ serve as a way for you to track whether you are being sourced from the unified field of your culture of loving, or sourced from your instincts in a culture of fear.

If these practices seem hard, if you are caught in a mental process of right/ wrong, if you are uncomfortable, anxious, tense, or breathless, it might be a good time to take a deep breath, go back to Chapter 5, and try some of those practices that are meant to connect you with you. When you feel yourself dropping back into yourself, then continue on.

Accountability: this is probably the most fundamental skill in relational partnerships that you will learn. When you are accountable, you can count on you, people can count on you, you can count on your partners, the Universe can count on you, and you can count on the Universe. You are here and willing to do your part.

Accountability has two very important components in order to really be valid.

First, you must be *asked* to take on the accountability for something and second, you must *agree* to it. And, you must *ask other*s for their willingness to partner with you for your needs and get their *agreement*.

This keeps us from assuming and guessing and running the world with our unexamined expectations of others – no requests and no agreements are two ways to get us in very hot water in partnerships.

Why Lots of Relational Partnerships?

Because there are no one-way streets in life – the energy is much more of a spiral. No matter whom we interact with, we are always in a giving and receiving expression in that interaction. We are either spiraling up in a culture of love, or spiraling down in a culture of fear. Everything comes back to us and leaves and comes back and leaves again. Even when we employ people and pay them a good salary, we are responsible for their humanity. Even if we gave them life, even if we married them, we are as well. If we choose a culture of love, we are accountable for giving to them from our best selves, sourced from the field of loving. We are the "them," the "other" and they are we.

Sarah and Stephen were both young professionals with one child and one on the way. Sarah was feeling the need to talk about how it had gone the first time around with the birth and baby care. She felt like Stephen had done a good job helping, but that he had never taken any responsibility for actually knowing what was needed. He never actually became accountable for caring for the baby unless Sarah handed her to him. She was still feeling resentful about that.

Sarah was looking for real partnership and not help. Stephen was busy at work and felt like he just didn't have the bandwidth to really dive in. He was just there when he was there and happy to help out.

Sarah was very happy that he helped, but with work responsibilities of running her own business it felt like she was in charge of everything all the time. She needed more from him than just help.

She really needed to talk before the new baby came or things were not going to go well. Sarah was already at a breaking point and already over seven months pregnant, never mind how tired and overwhelmed she was, she was still trying to be a great mom to their first child, Eliza.

Sarah noticed how snappy and unkind she had been feeling as Stephen whistled in and out of the kitchen, patting Eliza on the head, and sitting down in the living room with the paper. Last Sunday, Sarah had thought she might come undone when he asked her to join him for a romantic dinner.

Clearly it was time to get connected. They were able to find themselves in a conversation where they chose to really use the skills they were developing and look to see where there were things that Stephen could take on, and how he could increase his effort. Where was he willing to do that?

Sarah was able to speak from her heart and tell him how hard it was. He was able to really hear her and find ways to meet some of the needs she was expressing. It wasn't just things she needed done – she needed to know he was still fully committed to their life and to the family they had wanted together even more so now that there were going to be two babies. He had to look within and really consider it to see if he was really willing to step more fully into account-ability from his more distant "helping." Luckily, he was. They also decided that it was time to get some more help so that they would not both be exhausted at the end of the day.

They both realized that one of the bigger unspoken issues was that they had not had any time alone in weeks. Stephen was more upset about it than Sarah was and she was able to share with Stephen that she realized that she was letting her upset about the other parts of their life get in the way of their intimacy.

He committed to be accountable; to take on overseeing the gro-ceries and household supplies, and all morning logistics for Eliza once the baby was born. Sarah took on the hiring of the extra person to help (she did not want to give that up). When Stephen then asked her if he could take her out to dinner if he called the babysitter, Sarah paused, almost objected, and then realized that she really wanted the alone time with him now as long as she got an hour nap before they went. She wanted to do her part for their intimate connection and romantic attachment and she had to take care of herself first and the baby too.

She was able to go to dinner and do it without sacrificing her needs for self-care. She also felt immense gratitude and appreciation for Stephen's willingness to step in more fully, and since she had also felt met through the earlier willing accountability from him, she was feeling much more like connecting. She felt heard and cared for in his ability to take on more accountability and he felt heard and cared for as she agreed to some romantic time together. It is stunning how fast we can turn small things around when we are willing to be accountable for the state of our partnership.

Another important aspect of relational partnerships showed up in this conversation as Sarah was asking Stephen to commit more fully to their shared goal for a family that they were creating together. She wanted to be sure that he was willing to continue to be fully in for that shared mission. In relational partnership, another of the important aspects of the relationship is that there is a mutual commitment to a common goal. For Sarah his reiterating his commitment and actually taking on of increased accountability was very reassuring and important for her sense of care and commitment to her safety and that of her growing family.

What For?

This is the part that is "doing your part." In every partnership, each person has parts that are theirs. Your accountability is for doing what you need to do in order to get your part handled. And for giving your part of what others need. You will both determine what that is and how you are accountable.

And, in a place where people are often surprised, when you are in partnership, another place where you are accountable is for being willing to participate in receiving when others are attempting to give to you. It is much harder than you think.

Look back. Remember the last time one of your children was trying to give you a story, a moment, or your husband some attention, or your boss a compliment. Think back – was that easy for you to simply receive?

It is a funny thing when we think so much about how much we want appreciation, how much we resist it when it is at our door.

Embrace the gift of your partnership. Learn, grow, and become more and more alive each day as your intimacy and care become solid within a relational partnership of loving.

And, if accountability is not your thing – and there are some for whom this is true – then don't try this. It won't work out for you. Your best bet is to go at it alone or keep having relationships from survival. There is a lot of fun to be had but less likely a long term or connected commitment between two people.

CHAPTER 10

Listening for Truth

Listening and Speaking:

The First Ingredients of Relational Partnerships – LQ

One of the first skills I learned as a coach and facilitator was silence. After half a lifetime as the one all my friends talked too, the one who doled out advice, I was stunned at the power of silence.

My client Jenny, who is one of my clients in my transformational coaching program, called me in distress. I only take three clients like this at a time and I give them everything I have. My goal is to be there, their on-the-spot person, their *anum cara*, their soul friend. Instead of being there once a week, or at whatever interval we choose, I am there anytime (within reason for my needs as well) so I am available for these clients as if they are family. These are the fast learners and quick studies who want to be through the transformation portal quickly and on to their next learning.

One day in the middle of an important deadline for her and juggling a hurting child and upset family, she called me in distress. I attempted a few interventions to see if there was anything I could offer, but very quickly remembered my own counsel. I let go of the need to say anything, know anything, or offer anything, I offered the support I could offer in silence.

This day, I was aware that my role was to be listener. As she expressed herself with quite a bit of pent up upset, I was there to listen.

Listening in this case was and is an invitation into intuition, what am I hearing, what is being said, what is not being said. It is actually more of a listening into my self as I hear what the other person is saying. What am I intuiting, what am I hearing, what is actually at play here other than what the surface of what is being spoken?

Listening with love is a key practice of love intelligence, especially at a time when someone is sad or angry or just needs to be heard. I could feel her nervous system was out of sync, so I began to breathe a little bit with her, inviting her into a calmer breath cycle to bring down the nervous system response and invite her into a space where she could begin again.

My listening role was quiet but very active, I was very attentive, very loving and caring, and I was gently holding a healing presence for her as well. I was receiving from her all that she needed me to hold and then allowing it to pass by as I got what I needed from it about her life.

She was hurting. I was there. She could feel me present and available. That was healing.

I probably said no more than fifteen words of support and loving kindness, and then breathed with her again.

Within another three minutes she calmed down, breathed a deep sigh, and ran off to a meeting. Before she left, through her final tears she said, "Thank you," and then she was gone.

I knew exactly what I had been able to give her. She knew too. I certainly hope that everyone has someone somewhere in their lives who does this for them.

I hope you are inspired to provide this for someone and that you have someone who will provide this for you too. Bless you.

Let's talk more broadly about *listening*:

If you think about it, listening is a willingness to receive. And most of us ... well, let's just say we could use a bit more practice at that.

Luckily, we have a practice or two: it's like yoga – you need to practice, and the better you get, the harder it gets, but the rewards are deep and satisfying.

At the beginning of this practice I am going to give you a tip that in and of itself is not an easy task.

Listen with an Ear toward Innocence

Underneath it all, underneath all your listening to whomever or whatever it is, bring with you a sense of the innocence of who you are listening to. Begin with a sense of the perfection in what is already unfolding.

And add "What if there is nothing wrong?" "What if this person is innocent of my stories and my pain?" "What if I really listen and hear them?" If we really listen, we may just possibly hear their thoughts, worries, and what they have based their behaviors on. Maybe they are mistaken, maybe they are afraid, maybe they did something you think is wrong. We cannot free them to grow if we only hear them from the wrongness. We must listen for their truth and find our way with them to let go of any sense of our own wrongness.

Do we heal when we are feeling wrong or bad or separate? We have proven again and again the power of loving someone right where they are until they touch themselves and their own pain with love. You are the healing of love applied to their wounds and to yours. This is how we will heal and grow. This is how we will make our way to heaven while we're still here on earth.

We will love each other without exception. Our employees, our friends, our families, our lovers, our partners will know. We have given up the tight small world of right and wrong and will now be more of the solution for ourselves and others.

Listen from the Heart

This is simply allowing someone the space to share what is going on for them without interruption. No words. Sometimes it helps to focus yourself on silence. You, be silent. You, listen. Even on the inside. Really listen.

A word on *silence*: it is respectful, it is kind. It is unexpected. It is a powerful way to really see the people in your life. It will make you very popular. It is not easy. Silence scares us. It leaves a space of vulnerability. You will enter the space with them. Do not fill it. You will be tempted to. Do not.

Do this for you, your family, do this for your clients, staff, children, and husband. Just do it. Your life will be enriched.

Levels of Listening

Level one: Listen for content. Listen for what is being shared with you. Listen for what the person is trying to get out about their day, their life, their job, or better yet, the kids. What are they really saying? Just listen. Don't worry that you won't remember – you will. If you are listening.

Caveat: you will not remember if you are thinking about yourself, the time the same thing happened to you, or the list of things you still have to do. That happens to all of us all the time. The antidote is to tell on yourself. Be authentic. Everyone loses track now and then. You could try to fake it but it will be obvious. So just tell the truth and have them repeat themselves.

Level two: Listen for meaning: Keep listening in silence without pressure or tension. You might wonder: Why are they telling me this? (Don't interrupt, just wonder.) Do they need something? What do they need from me? And keep wondering – hmmm, what do they need to be heard about? What can I provide here? What have they said more than once?

Level three: Stay quiet and listen for deeper sharing: What is going on under the surface of what they are expressing? Are they unhappy? Hurting? Wanting to impress you? Wanting to deliver a message?

Level four: And when you think they are done, you say the magic words, "Is there anything else?" or "Tell me more about that" and then be very, very quiet. If you speak now you may never hear the thing that is close to being said because of all of your attention and silence. This is the place where the thing that they really want to say is hiding. This is where the hurt or wound or pain can be found. Waiting at the doorstep for them, the answer will often sound like: "It's just that …" or "Sometimes when you…." Often, their voice will be high-pitched or strangled. They are scared to say what they are about to say, but they need to. It is the thing that they never say and need to say, to you or someone. This can be a very powerful moment. Be still. Allow. Breathe. Rest assured, the silence will end. You will be fine.

Listen in Deep

You started out with listening to another person so that you would get a sense of what it is like to do with someone else. We are inclined to listen or at least pretend to listen to others' pain. And so now, listening is something that you will learn to use with yourself.

Your Listening: Desires

How do you know who you are as a person? How do you know what you like and dislike? How do you sense what to do or what you want? If you don't listen, how will you please you? How will your partners please you? How will they know what to give you, or how to care for you?

Your Listening: Needs

How many times do you listen to the crying of your children, the distress of a friend, the hurting of your husband, or the suffering of the world without finding an outlet for what is bothering you? In this exploration, you are the one we are the most focused on. You are the one we want you to hear from first. There are many *yous* that need your love and attention, the ones from your ego that kick up a fit when you look away from your needs, the ones that are scared or angry or still dealing with hurt from an old wound. They still need you, give them some time.

Listening to Your Soul

And how will you know yourself as a universal being? How will you know you are a universal being? How do you hear the still small voice that lives within you? How do you know your intuition or guidance?

In the deepest depths, there is the voice of you. The *you* that is always you. The *you* that can never be hurt, harmed, or endangered in any way. The *you* that is one with the one. The *you* that lifts you, heals you, and brings you home. The *you* that is the best you are, the you that lives from the field of love. The *you* you are proud of, the *you* you know you are.

We must get you home.

And the invitation becomes a way to walk through your day. Listening for love in all your interactions.

Listening to the universal support for you.

Listening with the question: where is the love here?

Where is the love in this conversation with you/myself or the Universe?

There is nothing outside of you. It is all available to you in the silence, in the quiet conversation within as you listen with openness and caring, love and power to you. The smallest parts with wounds and wickedness, the parts that love and care and hurt too, and then the part that resonates deeply in your soul. Come home to you.

Speaking

In this place of listening, choose your speaking wisely and sparingly, and when you speak, speak of love. Speak with love, with care, with kindness and gentleness no matter what you are doing, Be there with love. It will be returned to you.

CHAPTER 11

Honoring the Unicorns

Honor: Unique Authentic Sustainable and Diverse

The Second Ingredients of Relational Partnerships – LQ

Partnerships and life are ever-changing and ever-evolving. We are always getting a chance to see life with more awe and wonder.

We are one with each other as we honor our highest selves but, we are not the same as each other. We are not just like each other. In honoring the true self in each person, we are honoring life. Life as itself is diverse. And that diversity is what makes life sustainable. Conformity is an expression of our fear consciousness. When we are safe and sure of ourselves within ourselves, we want everyone to be themselves in the fullest exploration of how that is in their lives. This is a space of expanded creativity and possibility for all of us.

Everything else is a lie.

With honor, we are inviting everyone to show up exactly as who they are. In respecting each person in the authentic expression of themselves we are honoring that they are here in their unique form to add value and to help us learn and grow in our understanding of others and our desire to build strong and sustainable partnerships with people in every part of our lives.

And where that starts again is you. What matters to you? What are your deepest desires? Your priorities? Evaluate and consider, allow what is really true for you to come forward. Is there something that you have not shared that is truly you? Is there something about yourself that you do not truly honor? Something that you set aside?

"Secrets make you sick" is a saying that has been passed around by some naturopathic doctors and I first heard from Kathlyn Hendricks in her transformational Body Intelligence (BQ) work. And I have experienced it and seen it to be true in others. Not only is it true in our individual lives, but our secrets and our shame as a culture make us sick as a culture. So as a way of being sourced from the field of loving, we are an invitation to truth and wholeness for all who are in our midst. We respect life and every form that it wants to express in.

This structure of honoring all life and all the impulses in life gives the ultimate freedom to us all and gives us all a chance to explore life freely and find out our truth.

Be in partnership with life and choose something you want to support that is honoring of another in your universe.

What is something that you want to stand for in our culture? What part of life has touched you and moves you to be a contributor more fully?

For me, from my childhood background in the violence of war, since I was sixteen I have had my heart set on world peace. That has grown me into a very different person than I would have been without that desire. With that desire in me, I first had to recognize how non-peaceful I was in my life. Then, in learning about how to be peace in my own life, I have a much better opportunity to be that way in the world.

Being led into ourselves by a desire grows us. When we own the impulse to act, we actually have to become something new to fulfill that desire. I love that this is the way the Universe works.

What is it for you in the world today? Empowerment of women by raising strong girls, sexual freedom, love, God, fun, the environment, beauty, rollercoasters? What is it for you?

Who are you? And what does your choice to stand for and stand out about say about you?

Notice that some of these will make us struggle. Yes, we want strong, empowered daughters, but that may mean that they aren't as pliable and sweet as we would like them to be.

We want to be empowered in our work life, and at home but we are having trouble making both happen the way we have arranged our life now. Are we going to ask and create this for ourselves? Or will we give up because it is just too hard to make it happen?

Do you have a vision big enough that it is going to require partnership to unfold? If you have a partnership this would be a step into the health of your partnership. It could be to have a loving home, to make a new initiative happen for the children of the world. What is it for you that you both want to do?

To really make the things that are going to make life special to you happen, what new partnerships do you need?

What are you willing to do to be part of the new partnerships? What do you need to give?

What needs to happen in your current partnerships? Updated? Change of form?

Check in again with what your dreams are. Honor yourself. Honor your dreams. Look for the unicorns that will make you deliriously happy. Don't settle for an okay life.

What will make your heart sing?

Your heart race?

Your head fall back in ecstasy?

Are they in your plan?

Why not?

Who can help you get everything you want?

As we let our children learn about themselves, as we let them choose who to be, what to choose, what to love, how to love, how to express themselves, we choose a very deep respect of life, which always expresses itself in unique ways. Again this can bring us challenges and it's worth it if you value them as whole.

The snowflake is not the only unique being. No two of us are alike either.

And then, as we come together in partnership, we are going to have to share our intimacies, our desires, our authentic loves, our needs and wants and everything that makes us ourselves in order to be in partnership well. Authenticity breeds intimacy but it is challenging to be so open. Our instincts will want to shut us down. Keep at it. It is an attempt in the art of mastery.

At work, or even with your own employees in your home, if you allow for an environment where people choose the work they do by what they love and what they are good at, we find happier people who are more interested in what they are doing and will be more involved, more curious, more interested in forwarding themselves, others, and you in partnership. We will get much more individual contribution and willingness to participate when things do get intense. Freedom engenders environments of creativity in which new levels of possibility can be accessed. People stay bright and connected.

At home with your husband, find your way to give him space, time, and freedom to be an individual who has feelings thoughts and needs of his own.

With our children, our employees, our husbands, our friends, our families with shared responsibilities, we must ask these same questions above as you posed to yourself.

And then in each of your partnerships, once you have chosen to be each other's person, choose something to be about.

What will your partnership create? (You still have to maintain your partnership with yourself and them with themselves.) What will you birth into the world as a possibility because of your commitment to it and each other?

Make sure it is true for your partner as it is for you.

Is it a beautiful loving family, a great family and successful work, or a great family, successful work, amazing sex, and a beautiful life with your husband, friends, and family? Is that so for your partners??

We are often surprised by the responses we get. We think we all want the same thing. It is not so. What is it?

Don't let the how stop you!

This is no place for how. "How" comes in when we are scared to try something. How many times in our lives have we done amazing things without asking how? Probably every time we have done something amazing or miraculous. We are supported in our dreams and desires without knowing how.

And we must do our part but our part does not require a how. What is your part?

I wanted a family. I got very clear and followed my intuition. And I never asked how.

I wanted satisfying work. I started pursuing one thing and followed the doors that opened to me. I still didn't ask how.

I wanted wonderful fulfilling relationships. I started studying relationships and partnerships, and I still didn't know how.... And so on.

I have all those things. I don't know how I got them.

What I do know is I stated within myself that they were a priority to me. I saw it clearly, I saw the possibility, I wrote them down and fleshed them out, I found partnerships with people who could get me going in that direction, (some just came to me, some I "planned"), and I just started moving in that direction with those who would go there with me. And with lots of twists and turns in the road, lots of learning and caring for myself and others, I received what I wanted.

Now, that said, I mentioned earlier that world peace has always been a value, a priority, and something I have been up to. Some of my partnerships are based around that, some of my partnerships include that, all of my close partnerships are an effort to achieve that in my life within me, and, I have not made it happen outside me yet. I am committed, so I keep going toward my goal.

> *"Do not be daunted by the enormity of the world's grief.*
> *Do justly now. Love mercy, now. Walk humbly, now.*
> *You are not obligated to complete the work,*
> *But neither are you free to abandon it."*
> – The Talmud

The "how" holds the power to stop you. It can be a little side trip fear will take you on to stop you from making any forward progress.

Head for the "what" and keep working on your partnerships to support you, with everyone's well-being always cared for.

Guidelines for honoring the other:

If it doesn't work for one person, it doesn't work.

If someone is compromising, it doesn't work.

If someone is sacrificing themselves, it doesn't work.

Freedom is power and is a cornerstone of relational partnerships.

If you can't say no, you can't say yes. You must be free. If your partners are coerced, demanded, paid but not cared for or seduced for their allegiance to you and your desires, you will struggle. They must choose in freely for themselves.

And if they say no, you must respect it. You can ask if there is flexibility but be careful you aren't setting them up for your favorite manipulation.

And you can make deals with each other for ways that you can support each other's needs and desires, but it is slippery and often works better if you have some support. Getting support as you get all this in place is a great idea.

This can be a big shift for people who only know how to get things done by powering over others, manipulating, threatening, and betraying others.

What would our worlds be like if we all had this sense of honoring ourselves, our passions, our truths, and our lives, and learned how to work together to get great results for everyone?

Sounds delicious.

Angie was mid-career and a powerful member of the partnership at work. She was smart and quick and loved the chess game that her job was. She had proven over four years that she was a capable and integral member of the team and she loved working with her team in corporate training. In the fourth year of the partnership, the business started to change and the structure of the leadership needed to respond. Angie got scared. She noticed that she was thinking negatively about what would happen to her in the restructuring. She noticed that she was engaging with the other partners less and less, but the pressure of distancing was making her dread coming to work. She decided at the very least she needed to share her concerns and her ideas with the others. It was a big risk. She wasn't sure how it was going to fly. But she couldn't take the distance anymore. Anything would be better than this.

This team had cultivated an environment of honor, respect, integrity, diversity, and kindness, so she decided to take the chance and trust. When she decided to bring her full self out into the open and share with the others, she was very relieved. As she opened up and shared about her concerns and the changes in her personal life, that she was pregnant and thinking about wanting to work from home, there was a sense of relief in the room. As she shared, the others shared as well.

Over the next four weeks, the team met many times, each time each person bringing their truth and what they needed. One person wanted to move but stay in some form with the company, one person wanted to retain the leadership. She ended up with a pay cut but, to her happiness, the ability to work at home and work fewer hours once the baby came. She was also free to use her contacts and build her own business outside the day-to-day work of the company.

It wasn't an easy process, and her loved ones had some concerns along the way, but in the end she was able to work about a third less, and from home pick up some new clients along the way. Before the baby was born she was back to her salary level, working from home and happy and fulfilled in her work.

She would not have ever been able to achieve any of that without honoring what would truly make her happy, what her heart wanted and without trusting the others and sharing it with them. She was happy, her husband was thrilled and when last seen they were nesting as they prepared for the baby.

The strength of a partnership built with this type of honor is that it will be able to handle the daily onslaughts of life. In addition to the accompanying focus on the other person, deeper aspects of this honor, we are building a partnership with its roots in the ground, its heart in the earth, and its spirit in the sky. This type of partnership needs to be grown into and tested as it grows. Once it becomes strong it allows for shifting and changing to happen without it dislodging the foundation, breaking its heart, or losing its spirit.

As you are creating partnerships, it is one of the most important things we can do to have the people who are with us feel honored by us. What it takes to make that happen is not simple but as you apply that sense of honor to yourself, you see the importance of the components that we are calling out here.

Honoring another is calling forward their spirit. It is the honoring that which is truly unique it is the entering into a sacred agreement with them that they are divine and are also a valuable member of the partnership. Each of us are so unique that to call forward someone's spirit is to ultimately make them truly at home.

Your spirit is your tether to the natural world. It is who you were before who you are now. It comes forward with you and it is a powerful representative of you.

Ask these questions of yourself from your connection to source. You will go through these questions three times with your partner as you connect with the three areas of your personal culture; your life in your relationship with the Universe, with yourself, and with the other.

- How will you feel most honored?
- What will invite you into your truest essence to be in partnership?
- What part of you is showing up that doesn't always come forward?

When we call out the importance of respect, we allow others to come into our world with a deep sense of being who they are, beyond any of their giving, is accepted and desired in our world and on the team.

- How can we show you our deepest respect?
- What is in your personal culture that you know will give you a sense of the truth of that?
- What will you bring when you feel our respect?

In calling forward your integrity, we are inviting you into a team, a partnership that is knowledgeable about itself. A team that pauses to ask itself questions about its direction, and cares when even one member of the partnership is not in alignment. We are building a team that we want to have last and so we will be inviting each of us to be in an ongoing conversation about each decision that is made each path we take, each way that we turn on our path together.

- What type of support do you need for your integrity to flourish in our partnership?
- What can you offer that will continue to invite you into an ongoing inquiry with yourself and your knowing?
- What will you do if we get to an impasse?

In saying that we are desiring diversity, we are making who they are, their unique heritage, their unique whole self an important part of what we are honoring. We are saying that we welcome who you are, the unique destiny that brought you to this place with all of your background, and all of the ways you are unique because of that. We celebrate that you are bringing us a gift we would not otherwise have in our midst. You are bringing something that doesn't exist here before you come, and will not exist if you leave. You are important as we craft our tapestry. Thank you for being with us.

- How can we encourage you to fully bring every aspect of your fullness here?
- What will support you the best in your being in discovery of who you are every day?
- How will you let us celebrate you? What do you love the most to be celebrated for?

And in kindness we are requesting a true sense of attention to your truest answers, the thoughts behind the thoughts, that which you might not say. We do know that in the creation of this powerful partnership, we want someone who will speak straight with us. Share with clarity and with power, with love for us, while they share a differing point of view or a concern or worry. You will be saving us from our self-delusion. We want our partnerships to be strong and be able to withstand whatever concerns are brought forward, whatever is in you to speak.

- How can we support your ongoing power and voice to be heard in this arena?
- What kinds of thoughts are the ones you might not be willing to say?
- How can we invite even greater levels of trust in our partnership?

CHAPTER 12

Seeing Your Magnificent Light

Value: Appreciation, Prizing, Gratitude, and Acknowledgment

The Third Ingredients of Relational Partnerships – LQ

Y ou will become familiar with the power of valuing others. This will inevitably invite a sense of belonging and care amongst people. You will continue to deepen your understanding of partnership as your field of understanding grows

There was a sense in my client Valerie's life that she just didn't have the experience that she was contributing in a way that she was being seen. She had lost her inner luster and appreciation in her world. This was unlike her. She was working hard and somehow she and her partner Dennis were missing each other. They were not busier than usual but something was different. She felt like she was on her own a lot and was feeling a little set aside. She noticed the little things that he usually did that she loved – her favorite coffee, a little special chocolate he picked up on his way home, maybe some flowers – none of those things had happened in the last couple of weeks.

The more she thought about it, the more she realized that she and Dennis had not been connecting much at all in any significant ways for a couple of weeks. As she was puzzling about all this, she reached out to me. It was lovely to connect with her. My clients are my partners in their growth and I love to hear how they are doing and spend some time at the edge of this new discovery with her.

As she talked, she realized that she was actually feeling a lot about this disconnect in her partnership and how that was affecting even her relationship with her sons. The boys were okay, but she wasn't even feeling connected to them. She noticed that when Dennis took them to the park, she didn't ask and wasn't invited to go along. That felt off too. Something just wasn't right.

And then she remembered. About three weeks ago, Dennis had asked her to pay more attention to being appreciative and acknowledging of the things he was accountable for. He was feeling a bit taken for granted. She acknowledged it at the time and said yes, but she actually had not done anything differently since then. She started to see what was happening – he was distancing from her in his hurt. He had not brought it up again and she wished he would have, but she was happy to have remembered it and to get to giving him his request.

She had a moment of a little self-deprecation, but we both felt that if she could stay in her own source, love herself and the one that forgot, that she would be in much better shape to celebrate him when she got home. She chose for herself with some fierceness as she was choosing against a self-abandonment pattern, but she was committed so she went home feeling lighter.

Fairly quickly she felt a lifting of her sprits as she thought about all the love and appreciation she had for Dennis and for the boys too. She called ahead and invited the boys and Dennis to dinner.

She made all the arrangements and planned to meet them downtown in thirty minutes. She called ahead and asked for a special table, grabbed some flowers as she walked by a shop. She got to the restaurant, ordered Dennis' favorite wine, put the flowers out, and waited. When they came in she had taken the time to really appreciate herself for her remembering and all that she was going to do to surprise him, so she was very receptive and happy to see them.

There was an air of excitement and as the boys and Dennis walked in they were welcomed and brought over to the table. She stood up and hugged him and the boys, thanked them for coming and then spent the rest of the evening talking to Dennis and the boys about all of the things they were celebrating about Dennis that night. And, as she saw the difference it made to all of them, she made a note to herself not to forget to do much more of this daily. The effect of her kindness, her words of love and appreciation, and her sweet acknowledgments of Dennis' partnership were as empowering to her and the boys as it was to Dennis. There was a deep sense of gratitude and joy that went with them as they walked arm in arm home.

Seeing Value: Seeing the truth of who we are.

As we see ourselves and each other fully, we allow ourselves to see and value all of who we truly are and what each person brings to our lives. Seeing invites us into a sense of gratitude for the qualities that are unique to each of us and creates in us a desire to share our appreciation with acknowledgment of their particular contribution, inviting a sense of deepening understanding. Effective seeing creates a space of growth and action with initiative and vitality in a space of partnership.

Inherent in all of us, as close as our breath to us, is the need for us to be seen. There is an innate dignity in us that until we are seen doesn't really thrive. We can be there, we can even participate, but until we are actually seen and actually acknowledged for who we are, we are not present.

That presence is everything. It is in being seen that our deep sense of need for connection gets satisfied. Seeing each person and the unique qualities that they bring to each moment, each day, to each interaction is integral to their seeing of themselves.

We know that when children are not seen and acknowledged for who they are, they don't do as well. The same is true of us at any age. Being seen, really seen, is a gift that we give to others every day. It is the gift of our attention that makes another person have the sense of existence and a sense that their participation and collaboration in the whole matters.

When we are too busy to stop and talk to those who care for us or those we care for we are not caring for their whole selves. Stopping, noticing, and connecting creates an atmosphere of mutual caring and kindness that allows those who are around us to feel strengthened by our attention.

When we pause, slow down, and see each individual in our lives, we begin to see the richness around us. Our employees, friends, families, helpers feel seen, we notice the beauty of each life, the sense of the absolute joy of having each one of our people around us.

And as we expand our purview to noticing everyone in our day, we notice how many people around us give to us each day. As that begins to open us, we begin to feel the power in our world around us. If we stop and notice the number of people and their good will it takes to get us through each day, we have the chance to see divinity in action. We have the chance to acknowledge the inherent beauty in each being, in each tree we walk by, in each eye we look in.

We are interacting with life. It is pure beauty to interact seeing life from a personal culture of love seeing the value of each being, and being with that as we proceed through our day.

And again, we start with you.

Do you see yourself, do you notice the qualities of you that bring you to this day? Who are you being that uplifts you? Who are you happy to be?

Do you value yourself? Who you are being that makes each day worthwhile?

Do you take a moment to thank yourself for showing yourself to your world?

Do you breathe, look in your eyes and love yourself?

You are worth the time and it is a good thing to do to have these powerful interactions with yourself each day. Taking a moment to really see who you are will give you the gifts of loving for yourself each day.

To really feel the impact of this, take a moment and think about how it would feel if you got up each morning with a partner who stopped their forward motion when they saw you and looked deeply into your eyes. And then they saw you and shared with you the beauty they see in you, the light they see in your eyes, the power that you share, and the gift that you are just by being you. And then with deep reverence they shared their love and care of who you are and what you are up to and how deeply you impact their life each day.

Now close your eyes and feel that.

With this kind of acknowledgement, we feel a sense of a coming alive in us and rush of energy and a desire to step fully into who we are and what we're up to in our lives.

Seeing is a powerful gift of love to yourself. It will fuel you, fill you, and prepare you to make your life full of love each day.

We are all looking for someone who will single us out, make us feel special, and bring us to a sense of the glory and the beauty of who we are each day.

In giving this to ourselves, we are taking the power to create back each day. We are starting ourselves out with a dose of self-acknowledgment and appreciation for who we are, our *beingness*, which then gives us the freedom to be alive and free and fully available to ourselves and others each day.

You are the love you have been looking for. Sit deeply and still with yourself and make a big difference in your life today. The trees, the animals, the people around you will all begin to thrive as you move through your life this way.

Just being with yourself, just choosing yourself and sharing your love with yourself will begin the process of you being a beneficial presence on this planet, each day. If you do not do another thing on your list, the world will be a better place each day you choose this with yourself.

And then we turn your attention to the field around you. From this place as you notice life, you begin to see the Universe and how it is conspiring for your good, you can't help but begin to walk through the world with a thank you on your lips and in your heart.

You have become the love you are waiting for. Everything speaks its beauty to you. As you step into your day, you can't help but to feel the generosity of the world around you, the blessing that each moment is as it is given to you, and the wholeness and oneness you feel with all that is participating with you in your life.

And as this becomes more real, as you awaken to the reality of your giftedness from all that is around you, you will thrive, you will feel the guidance in the ethers around you. You will begin to become multidimensional, noticing far more than you have before that is here supporting you as you go through your day.

Once you have had this experience, you are ready to join the world with partnership.

Where are you being supported in being a gift to the world this day?

What do you need to participate from love this day?

What do others need this day?

As you approach everyone and everything in your life, stop, breathe, and ask yourself, do you see each person? Do you notice the qualities of them that they bring to this day?

Who are they being that uplifts you? What about their presence brings you happiness each day?

Do you value them? Who are they being that makes each day worthwhile?

Take a moment to thank them specifically for showing themselves in your world.

Do you breathe, look in their eyes, and love them?

You may notice that from here, not only will you change them with your attention and valuing of them, you will be altered in that same love. In the field of love a personal culture based in love, permeates the world and the Universe. The field of love is pervasive, all-encompassing, and beautiful. It is glory and the gifts of magnificence it gives to all within its purview.

Giving the gift of your seeing the specific beauty that is around you, within the *beingness* of each person, each rock, each tree, each animal, is the highest form of acknowledgment of the oneness of life and the power in the field of love.

Your world changes "the world" simply in your seeing in of it. Your blessing of yourself, your willingness to be gifted by the guidance available in the Universe, and your willingness to give your seeing to others is a contribution that will give you a legacy of love. Each being that comes upon you will be uplifted in your seeing of them, your acknowledgment of the beauty in them, and in your willingness to be a stand for who they are uniquely in the world.

From this place your love intelligence will cause your relational partnerships to thrive.

From this place you will see the difference you are making as each person comes into their own in your seeing and offers themselves to the world from a place of them. The difference you will have made is exponential.

From your personal culture of love, your life and that of those around you will be lifted, enhanced, and set free, to make this world a better place by adding the value of love and the power of each person's light into the world as the gift that it truly is.

From where we start with honoring, acknowledging, appreciating ourselves, we can see the magnitude of the power of the gratitude that is engendered and the good that you are being used for in this world.

Thank you for being you.

CHAPTER 13

Encountering the Empress

Empower: Accountability, Guidance, Trust, and Forgiveness

The Final Ingredients of Relational Partnerships – LQ

Kitty was always sort of a fly by the seat of her pants kind of girl. She had many interests and was smart and competent, so she took on new projects, learned new skills, and then moved on. She liked her freedom. She liked to have space to move around in. She liked all the contacts that she had and she liked developing new skills and talents. She was happy and contented for the most part, giving freely where she could, but not really stepping fully in to her full potential. Now, with her kids in school and husband away a lot, she was wanting something more.

She came to me with a sense of feeling the pull to make a difference in the world with her passion for people and the desire she had to help people get along better. She had a coaching certificate, an MA degree in psychology, lots of experience as a healer, and she lots of people who she had helped and cared for over the last few years. But inside her, none of that added up to her being able to make a difference.

She really saw how hard it was for her to take her contribution seriously. While she had worked hard and had a successful career in a corporate business, she had not ever reestablished herself in business. She had held some leadership positions on nonprofit boards, schools, and environmental groups. It all seemed like a big mash up of nothing to her. She couldn't find herself as a person who had any leadership to offer anymore, or any special capacity to share. She felt lost.

As we sat together she allowed herself to feel all of that, and then we started talking about what was possible in an environment where she felt cared for and respected. She was willing to play around with some ideas and accept some thoughts about next steps and what might be fun and fulfilling for her to do.

Over the next few weeks, we developed a plan of action for her. What was she going to do that would make a difference? How was she going to fill the gaps in her needs and understandings? We started to develop and plan.

She was coming to life in the exploration and finding connections and old colleagues who reached out. She was happier than she had been in a while and there was a little pep in her step that had spiced up her sex life with her husband recently.

Kitty was enjoying having a place to imagine and see herself growing and stepping into something she valued. It is not that the path was without challenges and she hesitated a bit in the commitment to a direction, but with a lot of support from her partnerships, she decided she could step forward and get in motion. The commitment was the hardest part. From there, she was excited about helping people through mediation and she found out what she needed to do to get her credentials polished up. Fortunately there was very little needed to polish as her other certifications and degrees were still valid, so she started to feel like there was something moving her forward, a bit of wind under her wings.

Her husband was happy to see her moving forward, and she was fun to have around. He was kind and supportive of her ideas, and occasionally offering his opinions in caring and purposeful ways. She was open to hearing his feedback as she really trusted him and knew he could be counted on to have her back.

She had a wonderful group of partners in this new venture and she was starting to move into her passion and power. As she was gaining success and momentum in her classes she stared offering small groups to women to empower them in their lives.

Kitty was very fortunate to have such a strong group of supporting partnerships. She was able to harvest their love and support as empowerment for her. She felt safe and cared for in her world as she stepped into a larger arena. She was happy and strong and well on her way with her team behind her, she was taking bigger chances and finding her way. She was able to begin to see a bigger vision for herself and see herself as a successful leader – she was even considering running for a local office!

Empowering You: As we work with our partners to discover strengths and hidden talents, we focus on safety and appreciation of their qualities to bring the creativity and individuality of each person out to the whole. We take on developing a culture of trust and ownership through accountability, guidance, feedback, and forgiveness, creating kind and caring environments with direct follow up for clarity and course correction, thus ensuring the opportunity for higher-level results from work, family, friends, and children in an environment of empowerment and joy.

In this section, we are focusing on what it is that we can create in our environment that gives us each personally, and that we can give each other in our personal culture of love, the possibility of being effective, strong, powerful, and getting the things that need to be getting done, done well.

We have listened, spoken, honored, and valued ourselves and our people, our world, and our universe and now in this moment we are going to address how we are with ourselves and each other that allows a way of being that is empowered to show up in those who are in our world.

As we step into the needs of the day, of our lives and of our work, as we feel into our desire to have everything flow smoothly and gracefully around us, we remember that we are the center and things in our world spiral and flow around and through the world we create with our people.

As we interact with our partnerships on all levels, we see the need to stand up and lead. Maybe we think we are not good at leadership or others are more natural leaders, and perhaps there is some truth in that, but if you are going to have what you want in your life, you first must choose it. And then, you must lead while empowering others. This will allow a natural unfolding of perfection. If we don't lead and empower along the way, we create a forced march toward a self-imposed end point with everyone dying by the road from lack of care and nourishment each day.

Ensuring accountability by creating empowerment in yourself and others is a much easier and more direct route to the life you want.

We think we know what we need, we think we know what people should be doing, we think that we know to walk an unflinching path toward a prescribed goal. We are wrong.

And once again, we are going to start with you. You.

As you begin this inquiry, a reminder to start in connection with source, life, self, and the others in your partnership as you set out to do what it is you want to do.

Again you are the center of your world. You are the center of the creation you are making called your life.

These are the big questions for you.

Are you empowering yourself?

Have you clearly decided the results that you want? If not, do that now.

Have you clearly seen the end point and really empowered yourself as the person who can do this with support from others? If not, do it now.

Do you feel a sense of mission for yourself and a larger mission for the world in what you have in front of you? If you haven't found the bigger reason, the deeper contribution you are yearning to make with this result, look for it now.

Are you fully on board? Have you taken the steps you need to take to make the space to create? Look closely at this now.

Are you choosing your direction with a sense of freedom and abundance? Look to see if any culture of fear has snuck in to derail you by holding on and forcing the direction to go.

Do you have the people, the skills, the resources you need to get started? What is missing? Yes, that. Go get it. Even if it scares you.

You are building an empire within a culture of love.

Are you taking the time to ensure that you are supporting yourself in being that culture of love as you go through this adventure? Setting up self-resourcing before you derail is key.

What support do you need for that? Do it now.

Do you see this life you are building as one possibility among many, leaving room for it to shift or change into something better for the highest good of all?

Are you leaving space for anything to happen that will support your larger sense of happiness, wellbeing, joy, creativity, and contribution for you?

Are you willing to be kind and create from that culture?

Feedback and course correction for you and your partners is necessary and a two-way street, and, sometimes we need space to hurt or grieve in the letting go, or change of direction or reminder of a need that isn't being fulfilled.

Can there be space for that in you?

Are you willing to stay connected to yourself in the process, to really look at what is happening, to give yourself a sense of your fallibility, your need to be reminded, or course corrected or even invited back onto your own team?

Are you willing to "be there" for yourself?

Are you willing to create powerful supporters with minds of their own, wisdom of their own, and creativity to give to your journey? Or would you prefer lemmings who just tell you that you are right and good and on track even when you are heading off to sea?

When the world you create is one of safety and encouragement, those in your world will be open, flexible, able to share the 'bad news' of failure or a need to change direction that may look like a crazy detour, you will have a thriving culture of experimentation and questioning, of enhancement and self-leadership in your people. When those around you are encouraged to take risks, and celebrated for their risk taking, and bring "crazy ideas" that come straight from the depths of their creativity, your world, your life, your business, your family, and your sex life will all be enhanced.

Creating a team of creative inspired partners will give you the chance to live a fuller deeper wilder life of your own.

Are you willing to live in the unpredictability of this world? While knowing that there is always a central purpose point of the culture of love within all?

You are creative, you are in leadership of this journey, but that does not always mean just what you can see. What if everyone in your world is encouraged to say what they can see? What if each person who supports your mission, you, and your life, felt free to tell you when something was amiss as they see it? You would be well supported.

And, when you are willing to create the banks of the river so the energy can flow in the direction of your dreams within the defined edges of your life, you will also empower them in the knowing that they will get feedback, course correction when where they are going is going outside of the course of flow if they bump up against the edges of your dream. This is your dream and your river to define the banks of. Those edges will give them the nudge they need to get back on course and give you the awareness of a possible need for support for them.

Are you willing to do that?

Will you do this for yourself and for your partners? They want to help. They need to know what you need in order to do so. And they need to know that they will be safe as they explore with you.

Can you be clear? Can you choose what you want? Can you see it? Share it? And create it together?

Can you commit to it? This is a big part. Can you commit to it. You must do that first in order to get anyone else on your team. It is your dream. You must see it, hold it, and give it away in order to have it.

And can you give your partners the freedom to add their own way, to be the "how" that you won't think of, to enhance their lives in the freedom of their own creativity?

This world within the letting go, this world where you can only see as far as you can see, is made safer and more interesting, richer, and more deeply satisfying for the shared journey that it is.

You are not alone.

CHAPTER 14

Becoming Extraordinary

The reason for all of the work that we have been doing is to put an end to all the suffering that is created in the world as we go about frantically trying to pursue the good life, or "happiness" from a place where it can't be achieved. After taking myself out in my career, exhausted and depleted from overworking sixty to eighty hours a week, my life has been dedicated to pursuing the real source of "the good life." It is my passion to be sharing all this and finding a way that we can instead, become centered and loving human beings who know how to care for ourselves and others, know how to bring out the best in ourselves and others, and know how to work well with ourselves and others so that we can come together to create a beautiful life for ourselves and a beautiful world for each other in partnership leveraging the love and support we have all around us.

What if our lives could be a gift of love to life itself, us, and each other? What would be possible then?

One of my clients, Ruby, called me a couple of months ago to share some things that were going on in her life and get some support finding her direction. She was feeling pressure and overwhelm from employees not pulling their weight, loss in business revenue, and her kids falling apart. There was something big in every area of her life. And, in the midst of our call, we were interrupted by her assistant needing to schedule self-care appointments for her. She needed to see the acupuncturist, the massage therapist, she had to get her hair done and nails done all next week despite all the chaos that she was telling me about in her life.

As this was unfolding, I was listening and wondering about all this. She is a lovely person and I enjoy her, so I was just considering what was happening around us. As she got back on the line I heard her say under her breath, 'OMG, my self-care is gonna kill me.'

And I laughed out loud. I repeated it back to her and we both laughed the next time. One of the biggest "mistakes" we make is that we think if we are "balancing" our self-abandonment with self-care that somehow we will feel loved. Indeed not. Overwhelm is overwhelm in any form, and self-care is not love. Love is love.

The minister at the spiritual center I call home in LA used to laugh with us about how much jockeying for position there was in the line for meditation. We couldn't help but laugh for the same reason. When how we are doing something or who we are being as we are doing something is directly contrary to the result we are trying to get, we are never going to get the result. The pushing in line to get a good seat so we could settle in for a peace meditation was as ineffective as over-scheduling "self-care."

This gave me the opening I have wanted to talk to her about getting her life on track from the alternate field that I have talked about here in this book. This is where our conversation about being sourced and creating a personal culture of life, self, and others can really change a life.

This path is one that many of us have traveled through overwhelm and over-commitment thinking to ourselves "soon, soon this will be done," but that is the fallacy. The need feeds itself in the realm of survival and instinct until we are worn down and run ragged at the finish line but we have great nails, brand new shoes a good seat in the meditation room.

But we are lying in the dust. This is where our story of overwhelm and overwork and over-giving and under-loving started thirteen chapters ago. It started in my life at twenty-seven, the day I walked out of my great successful job and on to the street in NY, free.

Ruby was finally all ears. And we began to talk. There is more, much more, but for now, the door has swung open and the listening has begun and her curiosity has been peaked.

It is time for us to let the love in.

Self-care is not Self-love

The biggest obstacle we face in life perhaps lands once we have chosen who we are, what we value, how we want to conduct ourselves, who we want to be with those we love, who we love, and what we stand for.

The place we will start with this is with our loving and caring for ourselves. We must choose who we will be and choose who we will not be as we build our love and space around and within us.

Once we have chosen, then the real work begins. And we must choose. The obstacle that is ours once we choose is to become the "who" we say we are, more and more every day. There are three stages that are not linear that we pass through as we spiral into our loving hearts, as we step into our wanting to be the best of who we can be, we step into a bigger challenge than we are anticipating.

Let's say at this point, we have decided that we are going to base ourselves in a personal culture sourced in loving, that we are going to listen, honor, value, and empower others – and then if you are anything like me, this story will sound familiar.

All these choices have been made inside me and I am on a playground with my two-year-old son. It is a big playground and there are kids of many ages running and playing so I am keeping a good eye on my two-year-old. All of the sudden, out of nowhere comes this eight-year-old. He runs by my son and pushes him over into the sand face first. Without batting an eye, my loving, caring, compassionate self is out the window and I have lifted this child up off of his feet and am yelling at the top of my lungs these words: "Whose is this?" – notice, no "child" word in there. The speed and power with which my nervous system responded to the threat was astonishing. There was no love, no consciousness, no kindness or compassion. I was holding on to the child for dear life, up in the air! This is the response of our fight or flight brain. Fast and furious could be its nickname. There was no space for consciousness, reason or concern. I was alarmed at my response, as you might imagine.

This is who we are. We are both powerful beings with the ability to respond with love and consciousness in one moment, and with no ability to respond with anything but fear and aggression in the next. This is where we must cultivate our evolving brains. This is where meditation, contemplation, and mindfulness begin to slow our reactions and reactivity and even give us some space between stimulus and response in order to interrupt some of our instinctual behaviors. Otherwise, even meaning well won't do it.

Self-love: Cultivating the feeling tone of compassion, kindness, and gentleness toward ourselves.

This dawning of the desire to be our best self (not our perfect self), the one we are proud to be, the one that is loving and free, is the dawning of self-love. It seems like it could be that this dawning would be based in our love for others, and in many cases people play it that way, but in truth, when this is truly aligned within you, when you actually have the best chance of being a truly loving caring human you are proud of, you must start with you. And when you do begin to deepen into the loving with yourself, you begin to see the love that there is to see in others. You are beckoned into the love you have for every other being dawning as the love for others, and then your love again begins to spread wide and full. And the next step begins to flow gracefully toward us.

If all we do from our love of others is open ourselves to the warmest inner embrace, it will lead us right to the dawning of becoming love. And from here, you will birth the process of becoming extraordinary.

This process of becoming extraordinary is an unending journey. No one actually really ever rests in that while still here on this planet. We have glimpses that are extraordinary, moments that are, experiences that are, days that are, and then we fall and start again. If we are lucky, we start again.

This is the journey toward our ever-evolving self. The one who is learning the language of the flow with life, with ourSelves and each other: as we all become one in the field, as we nurture and embrace the power we have, we still can't do it all the time. We will fail many times. It is in the choosing again, the recommitting each time to being who we are proud of being again and again, that finally opens the door to our growth and evolution and we are on our way.

It is in our most committed efforts to become extraordinary, that we can actually achieve moments of being so.

Strangely it also comes through failing and admitting that failure; we are not who we say we are or who we want to be all day each day.

Authenticity is our first line of power. It is humbling and invites us into coherence, an honesty with what it means to be human.

On a day when I feel great and all the world looks like love and joy, I am fully the me I want to be. Autonomous. Articulate. Held always and gently in the arms of the God that is me. On these days I feel the presence swirling in me in a way that reminds me that I am It. I am one with God and I am the creativity, love, and power of the Universe. I am a microcosm of the all and all the power is within me. I create from this space and all is attracted to me. I pray as me. It is my consciousness that I am altering in my prayer of aligned loving. Everything sparkles with the feeling of yes, yes, yes.

And on other days when some darkness is pulling at me, through grief or self-abandonment, through forgetting the higher truths or a physical reality that has closed a door that I was intent on opening, or many other forms of darkness that might pull me, on those days I am grateful to know a God who is bigger than me. The God that holds me on days that are like that day; I need that God to always maintain that space for me to get back to when I feel small. Without that, on those days I lose sight of myself. I see no future, no more days of joy and light and love. These are the days that sometimes some don't get up from.

On those days of darkness there must be something that holds the bigger reality for me. And on those days I bend my head and pray to it. I pray to something outside me, I pray that it discovers us and gently wraps its arms around me.

On those days, I must be still until I hear it calling me deeply from within again. I must be still or I will lose the one thing I can hear, the tiniest sound of love. I must not lose it. I must listen for it. It provides my hope, my light, and then a sense that all is well while all feels far from well at all.

I am humbled in this place in the loss of my sight and my vision. I can force it back in and force myself to embrace the power of the day. I can force a smile on to my face and effort into a gait of happiness. But I am not telling the truth about me. I want to tell you the truth about me. I want to know the truth about you. I want us all to tell the truth about ourselves.

I am sharing this here to claim my bad days so that you will know that I will understand when you have one. I won't leave you there demanding a shift or change in you before I sit with you.

I am not giving the others the respite they need in reality to have a bad day when all I represent are good ones.

How do they reconcile their pain with my joy if my joy is unrelenting? How can what is normal be normal if those who teach us teach us permanent unrelenting anything? You only have to live in California a few years to know how unrelenting one beautiful day after another can be.

Once I wrote a theater piece called *Have a Day* precisely for this reason. The relentless drive toward self-improvement can create a strain on our system that eventually becomes self-abusive. Can we just be, accept, and feel ourselves even outside our peace?

We can be more stable, or less stable. But, we can't be always stable. All gurus, teachers, friends, partners, bosses … all are human and all have bad days. It's okay. And, it's always going to be okay. Even on the worst days. It's just a day of forgetting our light, or a day of remembering our darkness. Nothing is truly different. It is just a day.

But in order for that to be true, we must be willing to tell the truth about our bad days. How else will we get the love we need from others – others who care for us when those days arrive? How will we know it's okay to tell them we are having one of those days?

How will you know of others pain if you do not allow it in yourself? How will you be with them if you cannot be with yourself?

How will we care for them if we don't know their pain?

Most if not all of us have been surprised by someone's suicide; some of us closer to the person than others. For me my first experience was with a young man and so shocking to me. I was a person for this child to talk to, but he didn't. Was I open to his bad days and his struggles and darkness? Or was I always wanting him to be better, fixing, cajoling, inviting him in for a smile? I am afraid I was.

But what was that smile hiding?

When you have these days, when you have healing to do, take a moment to feel your pain. Can you do that? Can you stay with yourself and heal those deep places of displacement and sadness? Can you be loving and free to be with what is with you?

Can you not have that drink, not binge watch that show, not have that workout that makes it all go away? Can you not rush to change your mind? Can you wait in it for a moment? Can you feel your self? Can you feel your pain and your own compassion for yourself? Can you give that to yourself? And can you love yourSelf in your weakness and painful moments?

If you can, you will be more real. You will be more whole. You will be more compassionate and be more resourced as a human and you will have something to offer others who are in their pain, not a commiserating in a story, just love to surround them and comfort them as they go. And then you will also find yourself to be more divine.

If we don't know how to be with ourselves, we won't know how to be with each other. And then one day we will be surprised. We will miss something important in our child's eyes, our friend's shaking hand, a quiver in our husband's voice, we will miss each other's pain, and we will miss the opportunity to share in it with them and restore their love.

Once we can embrace ourselves with love, once we feel the power of who we are and that we can sit with our pain until we are ready to lift ourselves patiently into the light, once the darkness recedes naturally in love, we see that not only can we get through this with ourselves, we can get through any of these times with our friends our loved ones, and even complete strangers. We are strong and holy, sacred, and beautiful when we are one people united together in love.

This is the source of being you that you seek. Sit in it and let it guide you.

Self-care, Self-love in Action: Creating, Maintaining, Sustaining, and Clearing the Temple of the Empress that is You

Am I full?

Beyond the love that we need, we need to know exactly what we each need to create a happy life, a successful life, and a life that we are happy to be living. And, we need to be able to access our power when it is time to stand in it. We are consolidating our power within ourselves by strengthening our structures, healing our wounds, caring for ourselves and knowing when to press forward with a fierceness that is assertive and not aggressive and invites a stop to an out of integrity energy in our field. We must maintain ourselves and learn the art of self care and self honoring so deep that we teach others how to treat us.

We must build a life with several components of care to keep us as close to our center so that we can have access to or live in our field of love. And we must find a way to create our stability. If we have accessed the field of love but we are pulled out of it every time something happens, we are at a serious disadvantage in life. We must support ourselves so that we are able to stand tall even in powerful expressions of energy from others. We can do this. We are strong enough. We must learn to consolidate our power and not collapse into someone else's desire to control or undermine us.

The Challenge

This is the great challenge point. We feel as if others' actions, words, and thoughts pull us out of our loving. We feel as if we have no control over our reactions to others. We feel as if we are justified in our anger and our emotionality if others have been rude or hurt us.

What if the truth is that nothing outside you actually can hurt you? Many of you will find this to be the challenge that I said it is. It is a challenge, that's why I used that word.

What if, no matter what, you are the only one who is in charge of how you feel? What if you are the only one who can stay whole in a situation where something intense is happening? What if, you together with your source, in a life where you are caring for yourself, are strong enough to say what is true calmly and with power and strength without collapsing into powerlessness?

What if you have all the power in you to care for yourself and allow what is not for you to simply pass out of your life.

My client Michelle was a very capable, strong, and powerful woman in some ways, but in her business, when one of the other partners would approach her with some upset, she would cave in. It was a place of deep frustration for her. She knew exactly what needed to be said, but she wouldn't stand up to them, and she knew that she was an easy target for that reason. It was like they could feel it.

They could feel it. Michelle's power was not centered in her, she was vulnerable to people taking what they could. In her business life, it felt like she had no dignity left at the end of some days. And she was so angry at herself.

We worked together with these different questions until she unearthed a memory of an old hurt between her and a seventh-grade teacher where she had been humiliated in front of a class. She vowed never to do that again, and so every time she tried to speak up that old memory surfaced in her body to keep her quiet. We did some healing work on it and once she had worked with it a few times she felt a sense of release in her body. She took her healing homework with her to continue to release the shame and sting of that memory. And to reinforce her healing as she went about her day.

In addition, she went back and looked at what she had created for her space to make sure that she had created a space that served her in feeling full and powerful.

Once the space was clear from her healing, she took on the hard work of reminding herself that she was powerful and was capable of holding her space. The healing definitely made a difference, feeling more powerful she first took on just keeping her self feeling whole, and eventually started even speaking up from her wholeness when she felt that she wasn't happy with what was being said or what was being dropped at her feet.

Her personal experience of her power was a whole new experience for her. She was able to see and imagine herself as more successful and in charge of herself, and she began speaking her truth and stepping into her leadership role more and more.

This shift is not an easy one. It takes a certain kind of vigilance to feel as soon as we feel the wind going out of our sails and coming back in to fill them up again. As we do that, we maintain ourselves and can be effective and calm as we deal with what works and does not.

Knowing what we need in each component of our lives is crucial.

This was such a game changer for me that it took me almost a year and three very intense weekends of trying to "get it" before I fully took it in. I finally had to learn it from a horse. Hopefully, you can learn this more easily than I could.

For this discussion, we will be focusing on our needs in central areas of our lives that are specific to us. I was gifted learning about this through my studies with Alison Armstrong and becoming certified in her work. This was an integral missing piece in my life. I had all of my spiritual studies, and my heart studies, my transformational learning, my coaching certifications and yet I could not count on myself to show up as who I wanted to be. I had a pattern of collapsing that undermined me every time I attempted to step out in the world. I am passing it along here to you with her blessing and with my own added perspective as I have used it and made it my own.

If you are anything like me, you have had this experience. You may recognize yourself in this scenario.

You are all set out to have a great day. Everything is organized, all things are planned, and then, something happens: your nanny is sick, the kids have a random half day, your husband has to go out of town. If our inner space is full and we have all we need to feel whole, we just pause, regroup, and move on. We may have to flex our day a bit and move the nanny, the housekeeper, the meeting, the date with your husband, or something else, but, it is not a tragedy, everything works out and usually even for the better in the end. You are in your space with yourself, you are whole and you can handle whatever happens.

If, on the other hand, you have sacrificed something that you need for any reason (someone else asked you to, you felt you "should," you thought it would buy you points with the board, people would like you, or you are feeling afraid about something, or you feel like you are alone …) you are most likely to explode or lose it. The less full you are, the higher the chance that you will bite someone's head off, singe someone's eyebrows, or hurt someone's feelings, and many times, irrevocably. We have all had these experiences, sometimes we get a little grace through an apology or the kindness of others but we must care for ourselves so we do not hurt ourselves or hurt others.

A client of mine named Susan lost her temper at her boss on the phone one afternoon. It had happened before, she didn't think it was such a big deal, but, within a few hours she was informed that her boss was going to fly into town (across the country and two hours from an airport) to see her the next day. As you might imagine this surprised her and she suspected that they would have a serious sit-down and hash some things out. Well, good, she thought, finally we'll make some headway on this issue. Unfortunately for her, that was not her boss's agenda. Her boss arrived, came into her office, and asked her for her phone and computer and asked her to leave. That was it. The company locked the door, wiped the computer and the phone, and left her in the hall without any of her files or personal belongings. After they had gone through everything, she was given a box of her personal items. She ended her career that day. She was senior enough not to be able to get significant work again in her field. It was a very upsetting and heartbreaking day for her.

In her sharing with me, it was clear that she was depleted in her life. Her marriage was not supporting her career, she was angry and frustrated every day. She was not taking care of her needs to get her life in order. She wasn't caring for herself at all and had slipped into a stance that others owed her care for all the work she was doing. That did not help her get her needs met. This event was devastating to her, her family, and eventually to her marriage. Everything she had built was lost that day. In her frustration, she felt she deserved more than she was getting from life, her family, and her husband. This strategy did not maintain her life. She took her frustrations out at work, she was flirting dangerously close to the fire outside her marriage, and she was spending as little time as possible with her kids. Everything that was important to her was getting buried under her unwillingness to care for herself.

We often see all of this as someone else's fault or their responsibility. Not so. All of this was Susan's to take care of. She was depleted and outside herself. The tool she had was to yell at others and blame them for her pain.

This is where the danger we do to ourselves lives in our lives. When we are not in ourselves, our pain comes to the surface and we will light someone else up even for something that could possibly have been anticipated. This is where we hurt people, blame people, attack and assault others, this is where crimes of passion come from. Something we need is missing.

In many cases, it can be as elusive as honor, respect, and kindness and when we don't give it to ourselves, we don't care if we take it away from others. This takes some looking within.

And in some cases what we need can be as simple as rest, sleep, a good meal or a great roll in the hay. But we must have it.

And in the end, often there is some of both influencing each other and leaving us vulnerable to our suffering and depleted.

We are going to stop here, and give you a way to sort out what these things are for yourself.

There is no value judgment in this. There is no morality or religion hidden in here.

It is a simple equation.

What do you need? Do you have what you need? If not, how are you going to get what you need? Don't pretend like you are okay without it. Everyone you love and care about, your employees, animals, and bystanders on the streets, your clients, your children's teachers, they are all going to pay if you don't take care of yourself.

This is non-negotiable. There is no way to get around this. Your needs are met or they are not. You are whole or you are not. If not, you must get whole again quickly. Period. This is your job. Not anyone else's. We will talk about how you can get some support for it later but first we must see what you need.

We all have a sense of ourselves when we are full, or when we are empty. When we are full, we will have ease being and accessing who we have chosen to be. But, when we are empty, who we have chosen to be is elusive. It is in many ways impossible to expect of ourselves. When we lose our fullness, when we try to give through the fear or self-denial of having less than we need, we fail. And sometimes we fail spectacularly, publicly, and heroically. But we fail. We fail by failing to be our true selves. No one is home. Our selves are gone and we are left with our instincts of survival to carry the day. We have seen that too often on TV, in the news or in our lives. This is the source of violence, anger, retribution.

An easy example of this, that we can all relate to that is not too extreme, is when you don't get enough sleep. Need I say more? I imagine you can easily recognize when you have a night when you don't get enough sleep and yet you push yourself to get up and do the day.

And now that I have pointed this out, is it easy to see how "you are not yourself" those days? I have been horrified at how I have spoken to my children (cringe), then husband, cats ... and what about other drivers, people "taking too long" or in your way?

When our needs are not met, we are easily triggered into our amygdala into our fight and flight system we have talked about before, and set ourselves on a relentless path of destruction as we fight, flee, freeze, and/or faint our way through our day. We are setting ourselves up to fail.

The emphasis here is on each of us discerning our needs, making a commitment to getting those needs met and taking action toward that end. Awareness of our needs and even the need itself is not always easy to see. Our needs are our responsibility. Going without is not an option as it puts everyone near us at risk.

Some of our needs are physical and immediate, as is sleep for instance. But some are deeper more elusive, the need to feel safe, to feel loved, to feel cared for. The need to have an impact on our world, the need to feel ourselves in some sense of interrelatedness with our world, the need to be needed.

We all inhabit a space that holds us and creates around and with us, the energy of who we are and what we are giving and receiving in the world. Imagine yourself in life with this permeable container around you. It holds your fullness around you, sharing it with yourself, and when you turn your attention to others gives of your overflow to them. When you are full, you are present and available.

As we touched on before, being full requires your attention to yourSelf in all these areas below:

Physical space. How does your office, your home, your car, your gym support you?

Body, your health, and well-being? Are you eating well and experiencing a sense of ease in your body? Are you flexible and able to be open and agile in your movements?

Is your mind clear and not full of old or negative thoughts and worries? Are your thoughts supporting you in forward motion? Are you able to think with agility and able to make good choices?

Are your emotions balanced and do they move through you easily or are they stuck and tamped down and in need of release? Are there issues that are filling your space with troubled feelings and misplaced anger, frustration, sadness, grief, or unrest? Are you in danger of losing it?

Are you controlled by time? Do you find that time limits you?

Are you always late or obsessively on time? Are you worried about getting everything done? Are you stressed by time?

Once you have identified what you need and paid close attention, it is relatively easy to get what you need. Most of us avoid looking. We think we can't have it, or it's too expensive or will be too much trouble or we don't really need it. That is a set up for a messy chaotic life.

And, are you here with a sense of yourSelf in a larger context? I won't pursue you here but where do you stand in the stream of life? How does your context support you in feeling safe and cared for in your life?

This is a wonderful place to be. Fully aligned with yourself and in your own choices you have the freedom to do what you want, live your life the way you want, and be the person that you want to be without anyone telling you to do it that way.

This is a great joy to many of my clients who have many times felt at the effect of others because they did not know that they could make some of these choices for freedom for themselves. When they grasp this and do it it is reliably a joyful experience.

My client Diana discovered after twenty years of living with her husband that she had absolutely given her power to him, allowing him to control the finances and the choices in their lives. She found herself having sacrificed trips to see her children, vacations away from home, and improvements she wanted for herself in the house and found herself feeling angry and distancing from him. She did not see that she had given the power away to him, it was very tempting to see him as the one who took it, but in the end she had to admit that because she wanted to feel safe, she gave away her power. She changed that dynamic, and was able to create a new way of making decisions with him. He did not know about much of what was bothering her when they had worked through this they were much closer and more intimate. She felt a renewed sense of interest in her partner and joy in his real kind care.

We are all tragically unique. The grand tragedy we play out is that until we are wise, we reject ourselves. But, there is no way around it – eventually we must face it and we must be ourselves. In order to have the life that we are meant to have, love whom we are meant to love and live in the center of the flame of Life. We must love ourselves unconditionally. We must deeply and honestly love who we are and give that out into the world with freedom. Then all that is like us will come back to us many times over. We must play the full out game of loving who we are and what/who we love.

A client of mine Betsy was teased relentlessly as a child. Her siblings, slightly older, would take what she loved and tease her, make fun of the thing and her attachment to it, speak to her with disdain and even sometimes destroy the thing she loved. And sometimes it was just her they would go after. She was a sweet child and often full of life and love and just as she was minding her own business, one of the others would make fun of who she was being or what she was doing. It wasn't until she was forty that she recognized within herself that she could not even discern what she loved and had no idea who she was as a result. She had such a protection within her against knowing those things in the off chance that they would be found out and taken away as they had in the past in the onslaught of her siblings.

And in many cases, the very thing that we are tempted to hide is what makes us unique. The way we be and do who we are and what we do is not like any other. To some, that will be attractive, to others not. That is not your business. Yours is to make sure that you are good with the being of you that you are and that you choose to support each day.

Once you have built your space you will need to maintain it by checking in with yourself and making sure that you are paying attention to any needs that need updating or changing in each category so you don't get behind in self maintenance. Just like you check the tires and oil in your car, you need to check in with yourself.

Our physical bodies are constantly changing so we need to pay close attention to how our bodies are doing, what they are saying to us, and what they need each day. The better job we are doing the easier it is to be who we want to be.

In addition, the physical spaces we inhabit must support us. Have we added anything or taken anything away that has changed our environment? Does it still support us?

If you do find material in the emotional realm you may need some healing and care by a coach or teacher, mentor or friend to help clear whatever it is and get you clear and de-cluttered with old stuff.

If you find some limited beliefs holding you back, you will need to go in to the mental realm and extricate yourself from those. Sometimes we look at our lives and see what's happening and then notice we have to look at and update our beliefs and our stories.

And again into the spiritual realm. How are we supporting ourselves to be conscious and loving in our choices, are we feeding the parts of us that respond to art and poetry the work of saints and sages? Are we whole here too? Or do we need some spiritual direction? Some guidance might be helpful if you are feeling lost or somewhat set apart from your divine nature.

Be clear. You are the chooser, not of the who you are (that is your unique destiny), but of the who you are being. Betsy's brothers were in charge of themselves and who they were being as those behaviors were established. Getting away with that was not an advantage to them. They may have learned some lessons later through some hard moments.

As we as a culture face into the effects of sexual assault, abuse, and misconduct all around us, we each must ask ourselves, who are we being with each other? Who are we being with partners? Friends? Are we pushing against boundaries or are we honoring and respecting them? These are all choices that we will each make over and over each day.

We will all err – when you do choose and then don't show up the way you want, that is simply another chance to be human and then you will have the opportunity to forgive your misstep within you and choose your freedom again.

Until you learn that truly the responsibility for your actions and your being are yours, you will be in danger of believing that others are the source of your choices. This is a very disempowering and deadening way to live. The more we believe ourselves to not have any choices about our behaviors and our being, the more chance there is that we will be at the effect of someone who does not have our best interests at heart.

And that is a dangerous way to live, because as soon as you give away your power, you are no longer free to be you anymore.

Here is the thing. No one is responsible for your behavior except you. No one is responsible for healing your hurts except you. No one is responsible for your life, except you. If you are stuck in the field of fear and acting out, or victimizing yourself, you are responsible to get help, sort it out and get on top of it.

No one can hurt your feelings without your permission. It is up to you to get that clear and start working toward that. Many people will argue with this, but no good will come of that. If others are in charge of you and hurting you and your experience is painful, you must come to your own aid. You must start by asking for help or stepping aside or moving on, or whatever you want to do. It is not someone else's job to do that for you.

As you blend both self-love and self-care with your choice of the source of being (the field of fear or love), and your defined personal culture, you, will finally be you at choice. Until then you are not. And until you are at choice, you are not free.

The obstacle that we face here, what we don't fully see, is that in order to do this, we are going to have to transform parts of us and parts of our lives and we are going to need partnership with others to do it. The biggest temptation is to think even after all this talk about partnership, that we can make these kinds of changes without investing in ourselves. We think that after spending years doing something one way, that awareness will guide us in a different direction. Awareness will show us where to go, but the getting there? That's up to us and up to us to support ourselves in partnership getting there.

We won't know how, and we wont know what it takes, but we will know very clearly that we can't do this one alone. It defeats the purpose of partnership to try to create it alone. It actually takes the joy out of the process to try to do it alone. Toughing it out alone was a costly mistake for me, adding years on to my transition, and depleting my resources, as I stayed frozen in fear. I spent years giving my time and my talents, but when I needed to invest in some guidance, I struggled to financially commit to me. I was sourced in fear, which is normal and the fear was making me small. I needed guidance for me but I was scared to give myself what I needed.

Eventually, I had to invest in myself. Finally I had to leap, if I had not, this book, these compiled ideas, would just be another stop on the road of non-completions, and dashed hopes. Investing in me pushed me right up against my sense of my value. Was I worth what it takes to have what I need to be successful? I decided it was important for me to do something different in my life, I couldn't create partnership with myself, and satisfy my desire to make a difference in the world without the help of someone who had walked through the fire before me drawing me forward out of my own way.

Investing in myself was the hardest thing I ever started doing. It has been years now, and now I can't get enough of it. This is a crucial point of success or not. And has changed my life ever since I have begun.

So step up. Own up, love yourself, take very good care of yourself, keep yourself happy and safe and live your very best life. Invest in yourself. Find the right person to guide you on your way and go.

Now, right now, you are being extra ordinary.

I am so very proud of you. I love you.

CHAPTER 15

Transform and Evolve in Love

Your future is love. Living from your love intelligence you will be able to be both at ease and expanding. It is the most formidable power in the cosmos.

There is a whole new world available to you now that was not even visible to you before. You have, at your fingertips, the process that can enable you in having it all, having your heart's desires fulfilled, and living the life of your dreams with you, family, friends, partnership, and romance, with everything supporting your life in flow.

When we substituted the world of love and creation for the world of scarcity, a whole new way of living opened up; a world of being where life is beautiful, and while still teeming with activity like the primordial soup of creation, you are more aware of how to be in life with all that is powerful and exciting, and all that you want to accomplish, without being overwhelmed by it so you can harness the energy and bring it into the world.

This is the path of the future. This is the path of power and strength of bringing your sense of your particular genius on to this planet at this time. You are here for a reason – to give the gift back to the world that you are. And to do so you are going to need these skills. And it is my great pleasure to have spent my whole life living, learning and collaborating with my partners and with source to knowing how to do this.

As we come to a close, the final aspect of this new way that we need to explore is how to get back to the culture of love when we eject ourselves from it.

In our environment, there will be things that will push against our knowing of our selves and the way we want to show up in the world. When that happens, what we do can make a very big difference.

There are many schools of thought and many different ways to get ourselves back into the field of loving that I have explored and I have found work well at different times and for different people.

Some are quick and painless and work when the issue is not too big, some are mental and some more physical and some spiritual too. This is the place where some of your other intelligences can help you out. Body Intelligence or BQ, is integral in reconnection often being the quickest route back into ourselves.

Within this book are some of the tools to use when you need to touch back in. Hopefully during the process of this book you have used the skill provided to you and are now more fluent in this language of self-support and love. Chapter 4 gives you clues on breathing and movement to restore you, and Chapter 5 gives you many tools of spiritual practice to reconnect you to your higher self.

Throughout the book, we explore your needs and getting them met. As you remember to look to your needs first, you can save yourself a number of bad outcomes. They can trigger us so quickly and then leave us in a storm of our own making. Addressing our needs can reduce the amount of chaos and drama significantly in our lives.

In general, if the work in this book intrigues you, I hope you will begin to work with it. And, while you could do it yourself, if you would rather have someone do it with you so you can do it more easily and faster, I invite you to go to my website and see what programs feel good for you. I am always available to talk and can be contacted through my website easily. This is the moment that you can choose. Would it be best for me to do this with all that I could give myself to be successful?

There are two programs in particular that I offer that pertain to the work of this book, beyond my regular coaching practice, and transformational coaching/consulting retainers. All programs can be combined and uniquely tailored to a client's personal situation and needs.

The program that allows for the greatest healing letting go and openness to forgiveness in my work has been the work that focuses us on what I call the seven seals, "Opening of the Seven Seals." It is a process that I have developed from my work over the course of my graduate school studies in spiritual psychology for healing old patterns that are stuck in our bodies. I have used it many times with myself and with others with the result that it creates a path where it is easier to be more present and more fluid in the realm of the personal culture of loving. The process is based in the chakra system that comes out of the Eastern traditions, and is a clarifying process which creates the opening for deeper letting go and healing, and the possibility of more freedom from our past. Sometimes when something we want just won't show up in our lives, we need something or someone to help us see and release a pattern we can't see. I would be honored to walk that path with you.

This is a deeply personal process and if I could I would put it in this book, but it is an experience rather than an easily translatable format for a book. It also includes some of my more individualized work. This work falls under the category of transformational coaching/healing and is mostly done on a retainer basis or on a series of three retreats over the period of a year.

It is a powerful healing process and allows for greater levels of freedom and power within each individual.

I also do this work with couples and partnerships of other kinds, offering an opportunity for real partnership to come forward through the healing of both parties. I have developed this work out of my awareness that the relational partnership work I have been doing is unique in its effectiveness and in the breadth of issues that can be resolved. In the partnership work, while sometimes it is necessary to take on individual issues, mostly I find that when the context is shifted the partnership begins to be able to do more of the work themselves. Shifting the context to the personal culture of loving is a quantum leap in consciousness and allows for all sorts of miracles to show up in support of partnerships.

The other program that I feel has the most direct benefit for the program in this book is below:

Raw Naked Beauty

Sometimes something very precious seems to arrive out of thin air.

And yet somehow as all the pieces began to show themselves years later, the threads were guiding us there all along.

Beauty has always been a mixed blessing in my life, from my earliest years of being a towhead blond girl in a Middle Eastern culture, through comparisons with my twin sister, popularity and not, I always felt hunted because of my beauty until I was able to find an eventual appreciation of a whole soul beauty through the eyes of other women who were not in competition with me. These women who cared for me showed me the way to feel my soulful beauty in my heart and find my empowerment through my embodied love for myself.

In first of many threads on this journey, my sister, a brunette beauty, could not see her beauty in the light that my blond hair always shed around us. My pain from seeing her not appreciated and not appreciating herself is the first strand of this story. I vowed to have women appreciate the uniqueness of their beauty.

The second was my own encounter with experiences of sexual trespass that happened, beginning before I was two years old and continuing to cross my path until my last incident at about thirty-five. My original light was bright and invited in experiences that made me dim it for many years at a time.

I did this program as part of beauty recovery for me. It is a deeply healing program allowing women to shed our fears, and self-rejection, our blame and sadness in our stories of sexual trespass or other wounds to the feminine.

In the year before I was gifted with the insight to share this work, I had two experiences that lead me right to the door.

One evening after a day-long retreat at a clothing optional venue, I saw two women I had seen earlier in the day now floating in a pool back lit in the night. It took my breath away. Both women with fuller rounder bodies were breathtakingly beautiful as they were set off in the watery light.

I am not sure I have ever seen a woman's body looking more beautiful than at that moment. It occurred to me that most women were more beautiful without clothes on them. I am sure that must have been the seed that was planted germinating in the soil of the exquisite artistic beauty I saw in that moment. That vision is forever mine.

In the summer, I wanted some naked photos on the beach of myself and I hired a young photographer for a cheap shoot. And I got what I paid for. It was dehumanizing, more raunchy than sexy and posed in the genre of the boudoir shoot. That experience cemented in me an unwillingness to ever have any woman have to have that kind of experience. It was good to know what I did not want.

From those two experiences, I was determined to highlight the beauty that women do not know we carry with us each day. The absolute sensuousness that is evoked in our nakedness, the innocence of our beauty as we let go of the outer experience of our pain and self-judgments and focus on the beauty we are that is evoked from the inside.

My healing with my beauty was brought into my life from many different avenues, and was deepened through the service that this program allowed me to offer others. I finally felt that I had created something out of my painful experiences that was in itself beautiful, healing, and restoring the innocence of beauty in women. We are capturing beauty as it becomes exposed through each woman's inner radiant light. A gentle peace sits with me about this process today, a humility, a sense of being used for healing for good.

And it is from this place that I offer it into the world. It is my passion, my healing prayer, and my heartfelt joy to walk this sacred path with women as they open up in healing to the beautiful treasure that they truly are.

For all, this program has healing elements, and a large dose of self-loving. It has served as a coming of age experience, an offering of love to a partner or husband, and a gift to oneself as a delight in the beauty of a body transformed through life, a memento of pregnancy, and a homage to motherhood.

It has been the ultimate confidence builder and empowerer of women.

I have never seen such beauty come to the surface as does in the women who participate in these days and the photos that we capture at the end of the day are powerful capturing of healing and celebration. They are exquisite, they are holy, they are stunning, rare, and almost unfathomable in their beauty.

The Process:

Raw Naked Beauty is a process of discovery for the client of the beauty that resides within them and how that awareness and the healing that comes forward from that radiates the beauty that the client may be struggling with within themselves. After the time of the healing and self-expression, we have a light, lunch in beautiful surroundings and then use a process that I developed called the "seven veils" as the client relaxes into her time unclothed with the camera. The seven veils are a sacred process whereby the client is in charge of her unveiling, empowering her in her truth and the extent to which the client chooses the unveiling to go. Each client has had magical experiences seeing themselves in a context where their true beauty captured and is seen pure and radiant from within. Some clients have chosen to keep their veils mostly covering themselves, some have had the veils off in a heartbeat, exploring being outside in nature and inside in a very private exploration of their own personal sensuous radiant beauty. All of my clients have reported having transformative experiences with their sense of their own beauty, confidence, and perception of themselves in the world. Client's demographics for age have been across the adult spectrum of twenty-four to sixty-eight years of age. For photographs and testimonials, please go to http://katherinemcclelland.com/raw-naked-beauty/

The experience can be structured as a one or two-day retreat, or have additional coaching with the retreat day at the end. It has also been offered as a pre- and post-inner beauty day for those who are making a conscious commitment to their beauty and confidence, a before and after. What is remarkable about these experiences is that the women's beauty is not more in one or the other, but in some ways enhanced both times by what was within in the woman that day.

This also is available as a couple's experience, retreat, or coaching package for intimacy healing and sharing, and it also has been used for up to three friends as a pre-wedding experience or families of mother/daughters. On a shared day photos are captured at the preference of each client, alone, together or a mix to the clients' specification. This program is a beautiful experience for a client to share with those close to them.

When clients meet me in person for a retreat, and it is desired, I also do hands-on work called body work for your soul, love and energy work that has powerful results as well.

All of these are further explained on my website at www.katherinemcclelland.com

It has been an absolute pleasure sharing my life work with you.

I hope you will be inspired to be sourced from love and a source of love and peace on this planet at this time in complete accord with all.

I love you.

My Love Letter to You

Love YourSelf

As you turn to this last page of this book, I beg you to listen. Not just with the cursory listening to which we have become accustomed, but with a deep commitment to you. To your own *joy*. To *your truth*, and to your particularities that make *truth* show up as you.

Listen deeply from within, listen like your life depends on it. Listen. Listen to your soul.

Wander off the mortal coil into your history, your lineage, your beautiful life that is yearning to be made free again.

Seek your *soul*. Seek your sense of your path, your journey, your lessons. But seek it not through what upsets you, allow yourself to heal that and let it go. Seek it through what you love. Live your love.

Explore the space that is you, the space that others will see as different, impossible, but you know as particularly, you.

No more think of yourself as common. For you are not. Not common, but also not special. You are unique, and blessed through the eyes and heart of the divine for your uniqueness. But, you are not more special than any other.

Every rock and tree, every grain of sand, every drop of water in the ocean – every one has its journey, each with a unique destiny, and a part of the collective soul.

You are the Universe in the particular. The more you seek yourself, the more you honor your divinity. The more you take your sweet deep breath and focus your attention on that which you love, the more you will sense that which you are.

And so you listen. Listen with a yearning to unearth the beauty of your soul, the intricate web that connects you to this earth and the eternal by who you love.

Listen to your people. Who are they? What do they love?

Listen for that which calls you home. Listen from the depths of your soul. It that you? Does that bring alive its offspring of love to the world?

As you consider, do not allow yourself to be captured by fears and noble ideas of what is good and strong and powerful to be.

You must listen for what calls you from the hollows of your heart. Listen for the dreams that erupt across the skyline of your life as you search for something more special to live.

Look for the moments of heartbeat and connection. Look for love.

Love what you love. Live as Love. In the field of love. As you. You are what you are looking for.

You are in the solitude you crave or avoid. You are both the listener and the listened to. Remember your voice. What is your sound? How does your soul sing?

When will you stop and listen? When will you breathe into your knowing, settle into your love?

When will you take the deepest breath of your life, open the door, and sit down in your own temple and begin? When will you sit at your own feet in the temple and praise divine source for the glory of you?

When will you stop running and finally instead turn and look deeply into your eyes, look deeply into your heart, feel the cadence and the strange beat that lifts you as you approach you?

Who are you to love yourself with such ferocity? Who are you not to?

None of your excuses will suffice, for until you do this, you will always be too busy, you will always be too distant, you will never know the secret of you who will guide you through your days.

You will be stuck trying. And sorting, and figuring things out, which as a life pales in comparison to one built on true love.

Your love of you is no less than your love of the Infinite. You are created in the image and likeness of the highest form of life, you are magnificent. You are Divine.

Embrace your truest destiny. Pass the doors of life that invite a cursory interest in what you like to do. What you like to eat or drink and ask yourself, ask yourself, "Today, who am I that I love mySelf so deeply that I praise the divine holy spark with each step upon this earth?"

Who am I to think that who I am is not holy? For what other purpose would I be here but to be a one of a kind facet of the unlimited infinite creativity?

So, for the love of you, love who you are, who you love, what you love, and that you love with a powerful reverence, a screaming sense of your divinity.

Claim your truth. And live your life of your dreams each day.

Gather your uniqueness like a warm cloak around you, create from your palettes, live from your joy, and bless the world with your special voice. Sing; sing your particular and even your silliest song. Sing so someone else will be inspired to sing.

Don't for one instant tell yourself that you are small or insignificant, because if you do, you will turn a magnificent universe of possibility into a jail and hand away the keys to someone you will blame later as having stolen your life.

Life cannot be stolen; it can only be freely given away. If you suspect that you hold yourself in anything less than your highest regard, then call the game. Because until you revere the sacred so specifically that you see yourself as the true one to answer the call, the true blessing to all, the true second coming of the loving consciousness on to this planet, until you see that each day is the rapture of your own world, you will not be *free*.

If you care the slightest for the love of the world, for the seven generations of love before you and after you, then resort to love.

You. In particular have an inner guidance system built in from your connection to truth. When your alignment is in tune, when your strength in refined with integrity, when your heart is free to land where it lands, when your world is safe with you in it, when life sprouts up around you. Then.

You will be *free*.

So, stop, listen. Wonder about your love. Bring the beauty of your heaven into contact with the beauty of your body. Let yourself express yourself with abandon, passion, and with purpose in discovery.

As we choose each moment to be alive, we will have no sense of what is next yet every sense of what is here to love. Every moment one question: what is here for me to love? What is here that my heart yearns to be with? Who is my love drawn to? Who or what do I love?

There is no more direct experience of aliveness than curiosity in each moment. Where am I guided to step next, what calls my deepest heart? What moves me now and now and now?

And, we must turn away from the lighter level of what draws us by its flashing lights to where we are drawn by our sensuous hearts.

Our love of our self never guides us in vain. But we do lose our way into loss guided by something we think we want, think we deserve or should have on the way.

This more cursory look at you will result in entanglements, in a sense of being lost, or unfulfilled or just even empty as we have forgotten to turn toward our self-reverence along the way.

You may do this life any way you choose.

Aliveness arrives in each moment, being chosen over and over in who we are. In discovery of the self we are that will unfold intimately within in its infinite possible interactions that are multiplied each time we land into a new awareness.

Is life an unending creative journey in the fullest expression of you? Is there anything more exciting, more powerful, more full of purpose, more divine, than you in each moment becoming you?

This is the walk for every life. If we stop walking with reverence for the glory of our individual nature and our individual love, then we begin to move toward dullness and stagnancy.

Even if your soul chooses a life of seeming stability, you still can choose with openness to what is new about you in each moment. We must choose to stop and stand into who we are now, breathe love, and move with grace open to the call of the next moment.

Who are you to love yourself? Who are you not to?

Be true to yourself. Beyond the desperately small sense of insignificance which can be nothing but a lie – look beyond and feel into the life that is you.

Fall at your feet in awe for the magnificence of your creator. Kiss the ground that you walk on, embrace the magnificence reflected to you in each turn of your head. Breathe in the beauty of life.

You were born to love.
You must love.
Or you will cease to be you.

Acknowledgments

A Deep Bow

These are my acknowledgments and appreciations as I am sourced from Love I know that I have never been successful doing anything "alone" – even when I was convinced otherwise. This will be at best an unsuccessful attempt in the impossible task of acknowledging and appreciating all that have brought me to this moment.

An Unfamiliar Eastern Kind of World

I would be remiss if I didn't start with my parents, Walter and Frances McClelland, and their deep desire to forge a new life away from the protected upper middle-class American world they grew up in. In our world away from all family and that which was known to my parents, my twin sister, Mary Elizabeth, figured prominently in my story for many years; between Mary Elizabeth, my brother Bruce (the closest to me), and my two eldest brothers, William and Jay (who even though they went to boarding school soon after our birth still remained the big boys we revered and loved), we were all we had. We had no grandparents still alive and did not meet any cousins until half way through my childhood. We were a little family seemingly untethered to others, making our way in an unfamiliar eastern kind of world.

And then remembering our wildly adventurous life, all those who contributed to me as nannies, helpers, and caretakers in the busy life in diplomatic cocktail circuit in which my parents were rarely home. Each have a piece in my story, some the kindest, some ineffectual, and some, sadly, the ones we were supposed to be protected from. The danger in my early years was both in and outside of my home. Unfortunately some of my biggest influences involved #metoo moments with those in whose care I had been entrusted but were not a reliable source of safety for me. The American Marines who guarded our embassies were a noted exception, undeniably kind, powerful protectors – even as we fell in love with them as we grew older, they were respectful and warm, caring and protective. A huge sense of safety, perhaps the only time I felt safe, was with them by our side.

Back in the US, a few times my life was deeply influenced by the political climate and the War in Vietnam, the death of RFK and Martin Luther King, the riots in Washington and marches against the war. All of my times in Washington were fraught with racial tension, with the retreat of white families and the bussing of more and more kids from the most economically challenged neighborhoods into the empty schools.

A Seminal Moment

This is when, savvy beyond my years, I read the writing on the wall of a bar bathroom I was frequenting when I was 16 – "fighting for peace is like screwing for virginity" – I was so struck by the truth of that message that I still to this day remember the moment I saw it.

My quest for peace began in earnest. Leadership in my church lead to connection with adults who mentored and taught me some hard lessons of love and life and trust. Bob Foley, Eddie and Lexie May, and Rev. Richard Miller all provided me with different and difficult lessons of life. I could disappoint and hurt an adult who trusted me, and while it was painful, I did survive.

A seminal moment to be sure.

In another pivotal moment, my best friend at the time, Amy Singer and I planted an imaginary stake in the ground for peace in the Middle East in our time, by 1981. She, a Zionist, and I, just back from a life in the Middle East, taking a stand for Palestine. Surely if we could be friends through this, so could others.

I have been influenced through some hardships, love and loss, war and peace by friends who deeply cared, kindnesses of teachers, professors, helpers, people I worked with, people on the street, and angels. Real moments, real angels. Eventually, I noticed, I was clearly not alone.

Beyond all experience in college, my learning, professors, teaching a rat to press a bar … boyfriends, love, loss, and peace, the love of my life, and that devastating breakup, influenced my life heavily. And after college, a brilliant group of never encountered before vocational education teachers influenced me with their care for their profession and the kids they were teaching. And in that job as a "teacher/counselor," my first loss of a child to suicide has influenced my connection to young people and parenting to this day.

My work in NYC after this – a radical departure from my path – was a fantastically productive and exciting time filled with the most unlikely characters, from a new best friend to a wildly inappropriate boss, to backstabbing and in-fighting and competition in the extreme, some kind men I was grateful for, some foolish, some just wanting what they could get, all of them were colorful deserve to be mentioned in homage to discernment and as a rather large influence in learning who I was not.

In my miserableness my sister gave me a gift that changed my life. She sent me to an Insight seminar and I was never the same. This was a second turn around of my life. I never looked back. Years of un-assessed trauma had resulted in a need for some very deep healing. It was to take me years and years, two marriages, two divorces, two step-children and one birth child, the loss of my sister and my father to eventually find my way.

On the Track of My Self-Healing

Thirty years after that first seminar, I am here today. It has been quite a life and the story I want you to know is what has transpired in my spiritual, emotional, and heart-felt education. The big early influences were those who opened my heart and showed me how to give back during the AIDS epidemic in NYC in the '80s. Insight seminars and their powerful loving teachers put me on the track of my self-healing.

Eventually, after my first marriage ended, I began studying the inward journey and the spiritual life with Drs. Ron and Mary Hulnick at the University of Santa Monica who became lifelong mentors and teachers of mine, leading me through emotional, psychological, and spiritual healing, after having first stepped into their presence in 1989 almost thirty years ago. Having studied with them many times and been of service to the University theirs was truly a whole life-healing journey for me. *A Course in Miracles* and Marianne Williamson opened me to a spirituality of love and an entry into the field of loving. Overlapping with that, Reverend Dr. Michael Beckwith (at Agape, LA) with Revs Carol Knight and Diana Trent (Ojai) nurtured my leanings toward the ministry after the death of my twin sister, and assisted me in the process of learning and leading a church over a period of ten years, eventually earning an honorary DD, Doctor of Divinity for that work.

Again, with some overlap, and upon leaving the day-to-day ministry of the church, my work with Kathlyn Hendricks and the Hendricks Institute opened me to the possibility of the healing available in the embodiment of my whole self, authenticity, and power of the truth that lives within me. In essence, it grounded me after a long period of living in a very spiritual realm.

New Generations

My second marriage came to an end and I was a single parent with aging parents. My step children and my son have had a huge impact on me, both in the parts that I have done poorly, and what I have done well. Of course, so has my second husband, who has been a soul mate of the deepest healing kind. I could not have done all the work I have done, had the clarity I have had, and learned and grown without the catalyst of experience that we created together. My family of origin, brothers, parents, cousins, and children, and the new generations of nieces/nephews, their spouses and children; my great nieces and nephews have all reinvigorated connections and renewed our family in the way that new life does. These are some of the most special people to me.

To the Morgan James Publishing team: Special thanks to David Hancock, CEO & Founder for believing in me and my message. To my Author Relations Manager, Bonnie Rauch, thanks for making the process seamless and easy. Many more thanks to everyone else, but especially Jim Howard, Bethany Marshall, and Nickcole Watkins.

Heaven on Earth

Within the last five years, I have experienced and integrated the work of Alison Armstrong into all the other work I have done, culminating in a mastery program that developed the strongest sense of my presence and my power integrated with my spiritual life, a true sense of living in Heaven on Earth – a goal we share. And in this moment currently, Byron Katie has stepped in as my newest teacher, my certain challenge to allow all of the facts of my stories to release in reverence to a life of loving and invite myself into the deepest awareness of freedom for me in my consciousness.

Through it all, I have committed to one friendship with Sarah Carr, without whom I can't imagine myself making it – my dearest friend of thirty years. Meeting in the earliest stages of our awakening, we have accompanied each other through all the ups and downs of this journey of life. I am enriched each day. We invest in our friendship as a partnership, we tend to it and it grows. I am blessed.

In addition, my life has been blessed by many opportunities to be of service. These opportunities have breathed life back into me when I have felt almost out of options and reminded me of the value I have beyond something I get paid for, the priceless gift of my love and the gift of love that I receive in return. Too many to consider listing here, but recently on the board of White Horse Wellness, as an empowerment coach at GALS LA, an oncology body worker for a cancer center, and as a mentor in the lives of young women in my community, I am again enriched.

In these last few months I have had had the pleasure of having my feet touch the fire of the passion that Angela Lauria brings to her work. I have risen from that fire and been given wings with which to fly by this powerful, wonderfully free and genius group of people who have supported me at The Author's Way. There is absolutely no way this book would have happened without Angela and my team of Angels; Cheyenne Giesecke, Ora North, Sharon Pope, Amari Ice, with special mention of Bethany Davis without whose support, patience, understanding, and flexibility, completion would never have come. And in the end, it would not be fair to not mention the crowd of supporters on our home team, I am forever inspired by Olu Sobanjo, Nancy Russon, Marlo Schmitt Andersen, Robert Heath, Erin Chandler, Ydalmis Carrasco, Ramses Rodriguez, Melissa McDaniel, and Meredith Holley.

Building a Dynasty within Me

Through all this, with an awakened spiritual life, I have been building a dynasty within myself of compassion, care, and love for myself and others, and for this planet, a reverence for life and for the magnificence of each life and the power of partnerships in the development of the possibility of peace within me and in this world. Here I stand a product of my intention for a rich and powerful life based in the power of love and a testimony to what can happen through letting "it all" go.

A deep bow of reverence to God in every form, every man, woman, and child, rock, animal, tree, ocean, desert, forest and sky and who and what that has brought me to this moment in peace to be a presence for transformation within the power of love in this world today.

All my love to you all. Peace, passion, love, and play every day.

~ Katherine

Thank You!

You are the reason for this book. My desire to love and care for you was my motivation to jump in and make this book happen. I wrote this book with you in my heart. It may not seem possible, but it is true.

This book is a book of Love, inviting you into the glorious life where we live together in the miraculous field of power, compassion, joy and creativity, passion grace and peace.

I am so grateful that you came here to read this book, that you drank the sweet nectar of love that poured forth for you. I hope beyond hope that you are taking some of these thoughts with you to implement in your life.

Please reach out if there is any way I can be of service to you. I can be reached most directly at Katherine@katherinemcclelland. com or you can go to my website KatherineMcClelland.com and contact me there.

What a journey this has been. My life has flowed with the generosity of Spirit, of my new friends and of all the mentors I have connected with and been supported by on the made this possible. I am grateful.

I am here to give back all the richness I have been given. Thank you for reading my book, I hope we will know each other some day.

About the Author

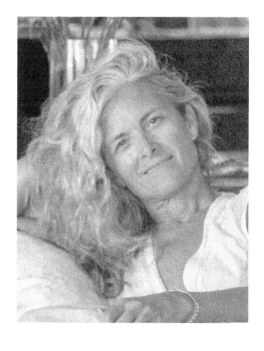

Katherine is the Love Intelligence Coach. She is a minister, spiritual life coach, healer, and beauty alchemist. She is a mind, body, heart, and soul kind of teacher and facilitator who speaks from the stage, pulpit, and podcast with authenticity inspiring us all to bring Heaven to Earth through living fully in our hearts and bodies each day. She has a BA in psychology; a master's degree in spiritual psychology with a concentration in consciousness, health, and healing; coaching certifications in mind/body and relationship coaching; and a mastery certification in partnerships. She is an ordained minister of Universal Spirituality and is also certified as a transformational leader and a healer. Katherine's business, Raw Naked Beauty, invites clients to see the radiant self behind their true beauty and captures that in the raw.

Katherine's life was designed to highlight the opposing forces of our humanity and to create the desire to bring out the best in us all. She has used every moment, every good experience, every dashed hope, every moment of grace, every moment of not belonging and every broken heart, to learn and now teach about life mastery, love, and peace in the heart.

Her formal education, life experiences, and inquisitive nature have led her to study new and leading-edge access points to being fully alive. Her passion for people and lives lived from a sense of the best of us, her joy in – and compassion for – our humanity, her deep connection to our shared divinity, her willingness to find mentors in the least likely places – all these have combined to provide her with wisdom that she now shares with those who want more from life.

Katherine's desire to know who she is and how she can travel her own life path in power and with ease, with grace and without suffering, is matched only her desire to share this outcome with you, too.

I Teach Power. I Teach Love. Requires Courage. Will Cause Joy

~ Katherine

www.katherinemcclelland.com
http://katherinemcclelland.com/raw-naked-beauty/
https://www.facebook.com/Raw-Naked-Beauty-Project
  -681011958577119/
https://www.facebook.com/katherine.mcclelland.18
https://www.facebook.com/katherinemcclellandembodiedwisdom/
https://www.facebook.com/holyfckpodcast
https://www.instagram.com/katherinemcclellandcoaching/
https://twitter.com/movebodyandsoul
https://www.linkedin.com/in/katherinemcclelland/

Printed in the USA
CPSIA information can be obtained
at www.ICGtesting.com
JSHW022332140824
68134JS00019B/1446